The Clinical Guide to Fertility, Motherhood, and Eating Disorders

This book is a comprehensive guide to addressing, working with, and healing from emotional struggles related to fertility and eating disorders.

Covering the emotional, psychological, and physical impact of anorexia nervosa, bulimia, and binge eating disorder, this book explores the lived experience of numerous women and men who have endured and continue to endure eating disorders, and difficulties related to fertility and parenthood. It delves into research on medical complications that can affect fertility, attachment, the experience of shame, and adjustment to the postpartum period, and offers clinical tools for therapists to use to support clients from a weight- and body-neutral perspective. Those who read this book will come away with a renewed sense of hope for recovery and healing from serious mental illnesses, and the notion that the value of having a family may be stronger than the eating disorder itself.

The only book of its kind, *The Clinical Guide to Fertility, Motherhood, and Eating Disorders* will be useful to practitioners, therapists, and scholars alike.

Kate B. Daigle, MA, LPC is a licensed professional counselor in Denver, Colorado, and has been a specialist in eating disorders, body image, and fertility since 2010.

The Clinical Guide to Fertility, Motherhood, and Eating Disorders

From Shame to Self-Acceptance

Kate B. Daigle

Routledge
Taylor & Francis Group
NEW YORK AND LONDON

First published 2020
by Routledge
52 Vanderbilt Avenue, New York, NY 10017

and by Routledge
2 Park Square, Milton Park, Abingdon, Oxon, OX14 4RN

Routledge is an imprint of the Taylor & Francis Group, an informa business

Library of Congress Cataloging-in-Publication Data
A catalog record for this book has been requested

ISBN: 978-1-138-54222-8 (hbk)
ISBN: 978-1-138-54223-5 (pbk)
ISBN: 978-1-351-00936-2 (ebk)

Typeset in Sabon
by Apex CoVantage, LLC

This book is dedicated to Natalie Grace. May you forever know the love you have brought my life and how you have motivated me to continue my passion to fiercely advocate for those who struggle.

Contents

Acknowledgments x

Introduction 1

1 **Overview of the Research** 12
So How Do Eating Disorders Affect Fertility? 16
How Does Male Infertility Factor In? 18
Attachment 20

2 **Conception** 25
Women in Recovery Who Desire to Get Pregnant 27
Clinical Tools for Working With Individuals or Couples Going Through Infertility 30
Miscarriage and Pregnancy Loss: Another Form of Infertility 34
Polycystic Ovary Syndrome 37
Secondary Infertility 38
Women With an Active Eating Disorder Who Get Pregnant 41
Physical Triggers of Pregnancy 45
Clinical Tool: Belly Stories and Acceptance 46
A "New" Eating Disorder 47
Clinical Tool: Perspective Shift 48
Considerations for Therapists 49

3 **Pregnancy** 52
Women in Recovery Who Have Experienced Fertility Issues 53
Intuitive Eating During Pregnancy—The Body Takes the Wheel 54

Women With an Active Eating Disorder Who Get Pregnant 58
Orthorexia 59
Clinical Tool: Metaphor, Meaning, and Moving Through the Mind's Monsters 65
An Unintentional Parent 66
What Would Mom Say? 71
How Moms Can Support Their Preteen or Teen as Their Bodies Change and Grow (and What Not to Say or Do) 72
Clinical Tool: Family Pregnancy and Body Image Genogram 73
Survivor's Guilt and PTSD in Pregnancy 75
Clinical Tool: Working Through Guilt to Acceptance 76
Birth Trauma and Eating Disorders 76
Clinical Tool: Letters to My Baby, Part I 78
Considerations for Therapists 79

4 **Postpartum Attachment and Motherhood** 80
Women Who Are Recovered Who Experience Fertility Issues 81
Attachment 82
Clinical Tool: Identity Web 84
Clinical Tool: The Power of Visualization 85
Postpartum Mood Disorders in Women With EDs 87
Case Study: Polly 91
Postpartum Attachment in Women Who Have Current EDs 93
Case Study: McKenzie 94
Parent-Child Attachment in Recovery 97
Clinical Tool: Letters to My Baby, Part II 99
Considerations for Therapists 100

5 **Shame and Perfectionism** 102
How Does Perfectionism Feed Shame? 103
When Recovery Matters More Than Being Perfect 106
Clinical Tool: Working With Shame and Infertility 110

Clinical Tool: Self-Compassion and Warmth Timeline 111
Pregorexia and the Effect of the Media 111
When Shame Seeps in to Your Relationship 116
Clinical Tool: Allowing the Pain 120
Considerations for Therapists 121

6 **What the Medical Community Needs to Know to Support Clients** 124
Infertility, Eating Disorders, and Privilege: Advocating for Those Without Resources 132
How Doctors Can Help 134
Getting Your "Pre-body Baby" Back 136
How to Create a Body-Inclusive and Accepting Home for a Growing Family 137
Considerations for Therapists 138

Conclusion 140
Voices From the Trenches: Words of Advice From Those Who Have Been Through It 141

Bibliography 146
Index 150

Acknowledgments

I am incredibly grateful to my family for supporting me through this process over the past two years, especially my husband Jeff who has been my constant cheerleader and stalwart hand-holder when I struggled with getting words on the paper. I am thankful for each of the brave women and men who shared their story with me for the purpose of helping others. Additionally, I am grateful to my writing coach, Amy Collette, and my mentors, including Marsha Wiggins and all of my grad school professors and colleagues who have given me the tools and education to become a competent professional counselor. Finally, I am grateful for each of my clients who have allowed me to walk their path with them, supporting them from a place of shame to a place of self-acceptance.

Introduction

When I was a little girl, I remember role-playing games of "house" with my sister where we would take turns acting out the parts of the parental figures and the children. It seemed so natural then; the role of mother felt easy to me. I guess it never crossed my mind that I might never have a family of my own someday, which I now recognize as an assumption I made coming from a place of privilege. I had a wonderful family who loved me and that's all I knew. So many others in this world cannot say that. This assumption that I'd get married and have kids someday stayed ingrained in me throughout my childhood and into early adulthood when I married a remarkable man. My dream story halted in its tracks as we began trying to start a family a few years after we got married and that vision of being a mother was ripped out of my hands. With each loss we endured, the thought popped into my head: Did I do this? Is this my fault because I had an eating disorder for 10 years?

Infertility, as defined by the International Committee for Monitoring Assisted Reproductive Technologies (ICMART), is

> a disease characterized by the failure to establish a clinical pregnancy after 12 months of regular, unprotected sexual intercourse or due to an impairment of a person's capacity to reproduce either as an individual or with his/her partner. Fertility interventions may be initiated in less than 1 year based on medical, sexual and reproductive history, age, physical findings and diagnostic testing. Infertility is a disease that generates disability as an impairment of function.[1]

Here are some facts about infertility:

- One in 8 couples (or 12% of married women) has trouble getting pregnant or sustaining a pregnancy.[2]
- A total of 7.4 million women (11.9%) have ever received any infertility services in their lifetime.[3]
- Approximately one-third of infertility is attributed to the female partner, one-third attributed to the male partner, and one-third is caused by a combination of problems in both partners or is unexplained.[4]

- A couple aged 29–33 with a normal functioning reproductive system has only a 20%–25% chance of conceiving in any given month.[5]
- After 6 months of trying, 60% of couples will conceive without medical assistance.[6]
- Approximately 44% of women with infertility have sought medical assistance. Of those who seek medical intervention, approximately 65% give birth.[7]
- Approximately 85%–90% of infertility cases are treated with drug therapy or surgical procedures. Fewer than 3% need advanced reproductive technologies like in vitro fertilization.[8]
- The most recently available statistics indicate the live birth rate per fresh non-donor embryo transfer is 47.7% if the woman is under 35 years of age and 39.2% if the woman is aged 35–37.[9]

More information about insurance coverage and the added financial burden to the emotional burden of fertility treatments will be covered in Chapter 6.

If a couple has been trying to conceive for a year but has not gotten pregnant, they will be diagnosed with infertility and will be referred to a fertility specialist medical doctor. When you hear about infertility treatments in the news, you might think initially of in vitro fertilization (IVF), however IVF is not the first step that doctors take to treat this condition.

First, a full assessment of both partners' physical health, genetic history, ovary and sperm function and health, and hormone balance (or imbalance) needs to be performed. For women, detection and treatment of thyroid issues such as thyroid disease and high prolactin can help restore reproductive health. Metabolic issues in women can also affect reproductive health, specifically insulin resistance, which can be present in women with polycystic ovary syndrome (PCOS) and in women with binge eating disorder and/or living in a larger body. The intersection of these will be discussed in a later chapter. In men, sperm analysis may be warranted to evaluate and rule out any sperm health issues. This can be emotionally devastating for a couple to endure who want a child so badly.

> My body is not working. I so desperately want a child but it keeps getting ripped away from me. I feel as if I have been diverged to a path that is full of thorns and darkness, not one that gives me hope or belief in my body doing what it was made to do.

These words from a woman who has been trying to conceive for over a year and is being treated with medication to help her body ovulate. She describes her experience as "shameful, isolating, demoralizing," and that she cannot trust her body anymore. Her experience almost emulates that of a woman who has been struggling with an eating disorder: the feeling of being lost, helpless, and alone, even though she is far from being alone in her suffering.

At least 30 million people of all genders and ages suffer from eating disorders (EDs) in the United States (with many more that have not been reported).[10] Eating disorders are qualified as anorexia nervosa (AN), which can be classified as a restricting type or a binge-purge type, bulimia nervosa (BN), binge eating disorder (BED), and otherwise specified feeding and eating disorder (OSFED). Avoidant/restrictive food intake disorder (ARFID) is a new clinical diagnosis for eating disorders and is not covered in this book.[11] These primary forms of eating disorders will be described throughout the book using the aforementioned acronyms.

With such high rates of both infertility and eating disorders in the United States and with eating disorders significantly impacting a person's physical (and emotional) health, what is their correlation? How are these two conditions related?

As I learn more and more about eating disorder recovery and fertility, I realize that I never thought about how my eating disorder might affect my chances of getting pregnant and having a family one day. I was 12 years old when I began wanting to lose weight. My mother had always been concerned about her appearance, and I internalized that to mean that I should be, too. Peers at school began to focus on makeup, trendy clothes, and hairstyles, and the vibe of wanting to "fit in" reverberated through the school corridors.

I remember looking at the way my thighs spread out on a chair when I sat down and thinking "that is gross. I need to have no fat on my legs, only muscle." It was the summer between eighth grade and entering high school. I was at an average, healthy weight for myself but I pledged to lose weight so that I would be "happier, more popular, and healthier." The big crises in my small world at that time were being part of the "popular" crowd, getting a boyfriend, and getting straight As—taking care of my body so that I might be able to carry a child one day was the farthest thing from my mind. I began cutting out food groups and counting calories and I dropped a significant amount of weight.

As a result of my determination to "fix myself," once I entered high school I ditched my good friends from middle school and set out to make friends with people I didn't actually know if I truly wanted to be friends with. I realize now that this was an attempt for me to soothe myself and my social anxiety and try to find some semblance of control amid a colorful and vibrant inner emotional world.

I have always been a driven, sensitive person, and as a child I often had a hard time finding out where I fit in. I was bullied for how I looked ("four-eyes," referring to my glasses) or how my name sounded. Kids can be mean. But I was resilient and made a few good friends and did well in school. My parents saw that I was bright and got me tested for the Gifted and Talented program, which led me to a series of special, accelerated programs during middle and high school. I was among the smartest kids in the city at school, and most of us were perfectionists.

Freshman year, I pledged to get "control," and I began counting each and every calorie I put in my mouth and cutting out fat, sugar, and carbs, as I thought that was the "healthy" way to lose weight. I had a magic number of how many calories I could eat per day, and if I stuck with that number I felt victorious, untouchable, elated—in control. But if I went over it, I was a "failure" and needed to cut down on my food even more. I was running an hour a day on an empty stomach, pushing myself to do tennis, softball, honors society, and drama club and keep up in my very accelerated and demanding school program. I was abusing diet pills in an attempt to lose even more weight, and I wasn't drinking enough water because I didn't want to retain "water weight." Basically, I adopted the opposite mindset of what healthy *truly* was.

What I needed was help, but the feeling of "control" that I got with restricting my food helped me feel like I was doing something right. Deep down, I knew that I was actually not in control but being controlled by my ED, but I felt so isolated and shameful about it that I did not think I could turn back or know how to do so.

I succumbed to all-or-nothing thinking, rigid rules that spanned more than just my eating behaviors, and I was quickly isolating myself from everyone and anyone. The more I became invested in my eating disorder the more it was destroying my self-confidence, but I didn't want to give it up. My parents became concerned and finally got me to go see a therapist. I was so resistant to talking to her that I said whatever she and my parents wanted to hear. I remember her telling me "you're not out of the woods yet" when I told her I didn't think I needed to see her anymore. She was right; I was so deep in the woods that I couldn't see the light of day. But I was still resistant to making a change.

My sophomore year of high school felt a bit more stable than freshman year, probably because I was adapting to the intense circumstances. I was doing well academically and feeling slightly more connected socially, but I still felt very uncomfortable in my skin and didn't know how to cope with all of the internal and external pressure I felt. I was still restricting my food pretty severely, although not as dramatically as the previous school year. Little did I know, my ED wasn't going into remission; it was just lying in wait until it could morph into another version of itself, like a shape-shifter.

I was on the tennis team at school, and I have a distinct memory of feeling so proud that I could fit into a size 2 tennis skirt. I just wanted to keep up that feeling, no matter how surface level it was. My self-worth became based on how I perceived I was being portrayed by others, an external locus of validation that quickly became toxic.

As a shy and sensitive teenager, the social dynamics of high school were extremely stressful for me. I now think I have always been a highly sensitive person (HSP), but did not know if that was accepted or okay, probably because the other sensitive people like me were hiding their true feelings as well. I absorbed the idea that sensitivity was not a desirable temperament trait. I continually felt rejected by peers and boys that I had a crush on (even if that was my own perception and not the reality). I felt perpetually more isolated, although I don't know that anyone would have noticed that from the outside. The appearance of "being okay" seemed so much more important than anything else.

I vividly remember the day I bought a large package of M&M's when I couldn't tolerate the deprivation anymore. I began eating them. They tasted so good. These were "forbidden" foods that I hadn't allowed myself to eat very often for the past couple of years. My body was literally starving for them. The thought popped into my mind: "You can eat this entire bag and then you can throw it up and you won't have to deal with any of the consequences." Magical thinking once again (thanks, ED). This is when my eating disorder morphed into bulimia.

I thought I was all alone. I was bingeing and purging several times a week throughout my junior and senior year. It quickly became a daily occurrence: at school, at home, anywhere I could find an opportunity to do so. It almost became a strange thrill to see how narrowly I could miss getting caught—"risky behaviors" that are common with bulimia. I didn't know much about eating disorders at all, but once I was fully in mine I was consumed with the complex feelings of shame, pain, and relief that my ED gave me. I didn't think that anyone else could possibly relate to what I was doing and feeling, and the behaviors I was engaging in were so secretive, so shameful that there was no way I was going to tell anyone about it. Plus, if I did, they may try to take it away. And I wasn't ready for that.

Little did I know that there were most likely a dozen of my classmates who were going through something similar, several of whom I have since reconnected with and we have shared our eerily similar stories.

I took a gap year between high school and college, mostly as a break from the intensity that was high school. I spent the first half of that year living in a castle in the Loire Valley of France, helping run the hotel and practicing my French. I loved it there, but it was also very lonely as I was the only American there and the youngest, marking my 18th birthday during my time there. I remember that my bingeing and purging behaviors stopped. I thought "I'm recovered! All I needed to do was come to France and be away from the stressors of home." I also missed my menstrual period for the time I was there and cycled into restriction again, although for many years I did not want to admit that this is what happened. My ED morphed again. I learned that year that the ED does not go away if you change your external environment; the internal environment can stay the same no matter where you are in the world.

In college I continued to struggle with bulimia even more severely than I did in high school. My friends noticed my secretive behaviors and had an intervention with me, and I realized this was finally the time. I didn't want to live like this anymore. I returned to the castle in France for the summer after freshman year of college, hoping that maybe I would cease behaviors again and feel better about myself. Instead, my bulimia continued and I was so ashamed that I couldn't recreate that experience I had had the first time in France. This is the lowest I had ever been, and I had thoughts about wanting to end my life. Instead, I was honest with my family about what was going on, returned to the United States, and went to my college counseling center and met the therapist who would help me change my life forever.

She herself had recovered from an eating disorder and gave me hope that I could do so too. It took several years, lots of outpatient therapy, an intensive outpatient program, and many support groups, reading, and journaling, but I committed to myself that I was never going back to the shame, guilt, pain, and disgust I felt while in my ED. It was like saying goodbye to a whole other life, a separate existence that I had been living my entire teenage years.

I was 22 when I fully entered recovery. I was mature enough to think about my future at this point and two of the strongest motivators for me were (1) having a family one day and (2) having a successful career. I also really wanted to find out who I was without an ED, as it had consumed me during a time of my life that was rich in identity development. In college I had entered an evening intensive outpatient program. There I was with many young women like myself, but also several women who were much older, in their fifties and sixties. I told myself: "there is NO WAY I will be still dealing with this when I am 50." The thought of that scared me to death. I didn't see any of the dreams I had for myself to be possible with an active ED. I also was just so *tired* of struggling so much and decided enough was enough. I was going to recover. I decided to dedicate myself to therapy and to recovery and did not look back. I had a couple of lapses along the way (which is a normal part of recovery; how else would you learn what it's all about?), but have been fully in recovery since that time.

After graduating from college and working in a non-career job for a few years, I finally felt like myself for the very first time in my adult life. I realized the severity of my eating disorder history and how much havoc it had caused me and my family. I also realized that having a therapist who had recovered from an eating disorder herself was so helpful for me—I felt like she could relate. I had a desire to give back and help others, and maybe help them prevent for themselves the decade of struggle and suffering that I went through.

I entered graduate school for Counseling Psychology and Counselor Education at the University of Colorado Denver in 2007 and graduated in 2010 with a focus on the systemic treatment of eating disorders. I have had my private practice since 2010 and have helped hundreds of people find their own path to healing. I am so grateful for my recovery and for getting to help others find theirs, too. My life has taken so many turns that I would not have expected when I was 6, playing with my sister, but I am where I was always destined to be.

When I was 24, I had been in healthy recovery for over two years and met the man who would later become my husband. By all external sources, I was physically healthy, stable, and recovered. I was a normal weight, I had regular periods, I was strong, and I had no disordered eating behaviors. I was also very emotionally stable and remember this time as one of the happiest and (truly) healthiest times of my life. I knew myself well and finally loved myself, although I did (and still do) struggle with anxiety and a perfectionistic, critical mindset that never seemed to give me a solid break.

I married Jeff when I was 27, and a few years later we decided we wanted to try to start a family. I didn't know anything about the connection between eating disorders and fertility at the time, but was aware that I'd been in sustained recovery for almost ten years at that point, and it didn't cross my mind that my ED past would play a part in my desire to have a family.

It took us almost a year of trying before I got pregnant. Those months were grueling; each month was yet another loss to grieve. I began having thoughts pop up that said "maybe you can't get pregnant because you messed up your body so much." I immediately recognized this as my past ED voice and quickly diffused these thoughts. None of my medical doctors asked me if I had a current or past eating disorder. I had to be the one to bring up the topic, which was uncomfortable, and ask: "is this something that could be affecting my fertility?" They told me they were not sure, but did not think so because I was healthy in every way they could measure.

I told myself what the doctors had told me: "You are healthy, you have been in stable recovery for many years. Those negative thoughts are only thoughts in your mind." I focused on taking care of myself with nutrition, exercise, sleep, and self-care, doing the best I could to set the stage for a healthy pregnancy.

In February 2014, I finally got pregnant. I couldn't believe it. We were so excited and cautiously optimistic about finally having a family. It entered my mind that it could result in miscarriage, but I didn't know anyone who had had a miscarriage (or so I thought—yet another topic that was not often discussed, but I found is very common), so I didn't think it would happen to me. We told our immediate family our happy news and my mind jumped to "I'm going to be a mom." I was anxious and excited.

In April 2014 we had our first ultrasound; all was well. Two days after that I began spotting. The doctor called this a "threatened miscarriage" and said that it didn't necessarily mean it would result in a miscarriage but to watch the bleeding. I kept bleeding and cramping, and then the worst possible thing that I could imagine happened.

Jeff and I were devastated. Our families were devastated. Our small circle of close friends knew, and were supportive. But then they stopped asking or talking about it. And we were just beginning to grieve. Jeff and I planted a tree in the place where we buried our first child, a tree that I still look at and remember daily.

I wanted to try again relatively quickly. I noticed some of those same thoughts coming back: "You did this to yourself. Your ED caused this." I knew they were irrational, but a part of me believed them and I felt so horribly awful. I thought that if we tried again in a few months, we could move past this. I realize now that my desire to try to conceive again was my attempt to avoid feeling the intense pain that I was experiencing. I did my best to cope with this in a healthy way, but it brought back such feelings of shame and failure that I had also felt in my ED that I just wanted to "fix" it by trying again.

We did, and about four months later I got pregnant again. This time I was almost consumed with anxiety. I was cautiously excited but more self-protective than anything else. We told even fewer people this time around. I counted the days until our first ultrasound. We went in, and the tech told us there was a heartbeat but it was measuring a couple weeks behind. Panic set in. I left that appointment in fight or flight mode. I was on automatic pilot and just going through the motions; my emotions were barricaded behind a strong barrier of self-protection. A couple of days later I began spotting again, with it turning into more heavy bleeding. I knew what was happening but couldn't believe it. I didn't want to believe it. I still had some thoughts going on that said "maybe it won't be the same this time. Maybe the bleeding will stop." Jeff and I sat there feeling hopeless and devastated.

The day that I miscarried my second child, I went tubing on a mountain creek with some friends as a way to try to get my mind off of what I already knew was happening but did not want to admit or face. On my tube, I got separated from the rest of the group. I got caught in an eddy, which is a swirl of water that just keeps swirling and swirling and never stops. It wasn't particularly fast or dangerous, but the current was pretty strong and I didn't have any way to get out or push off the rocks beside me. I sat there swirling around and around in the eddy for a long time, reflecting on how this experience was exactly like what I was going through in my life, with my pregnancies. Swirling in circles, not going anywhere. Stuck. The symbolism caused me to burst into tears.

The doctors found nothing wrong with me. After the second miscarriage I had many irrational thoughts about my past ED being the reason

I couldn't have a baby. I thought there was something wrong with me and that it was my fault (this is *exactly* what the ED mindset tells you). I focused on self-care and attempting to grieve. I was so angry, so hurt, and I didn't know if I wanted to try again. Deep down I desperately wanted to have a baby but didn't know if I could go through that again. I didn't know if Jeff and I could endure that again.

We took almost a year off and decided not to actively try. We grieved, we worked, we tried to move on and not have getting pregnant consume us.

In June 2015 I got pregnant again.

I remember the flood of anxiety and fear come back to me just as before. I was in that situation again but didn't know if I could survive a third miscarriage. I told myself that if it happened again then I was not going to try ever again (protective mode; I knew deep down that I would keep trying, but that the pain seemed too much at the time to even consider this).

We went to our first ultrasound and there was a heartbeat. It all looked good. This I had done before. I remember leaving that appointment and one part of me just expecting to start spotting. That is what has been the pattern to this point. I was again in fight or flight mode, not willing to let myself believe that I could have a sustainable pregnancy this time. Those first few weeks went *so* slowly.

Both Jeff and I were on pins and needles, hoping all would be okay. Jeff now tells me that he was bracing for me to come to him crying again, and watched me so closely and nervously for weeks. We were both still traumatized by our earlier experiences, as if the powers that be were going to take this baby away from us too.

I had elevated anxiety for the first 4 months of my pregnancy with my daughter. I knew what the doctors were telling me: everything looks great. But I also knew that I hadn't been able to trust my body before, so how could I fully do so now?

Eventually I became deeply attached to my baby inside of my body and was able to relax and connect with myself and my body. I slowly was able to shift away from anxiety, and into acceptance. I was going to have a baby. Finally. Pregnancy was a beautiful time in my life. Each body ache, change, stretch mark, and sleepless night I was grateful for. Well, the insomnia I actually wasn't.

In March 2016, I delivered a healthy baby girl. She is the light of our lives. As I have grown into the biggest new role of my life—mother—I have also reflected on my journey and the intense shame, fear, and pain I felt. I didn't know anyone else who was going through that (or so I thought—a theme in my life). I realize now that I was not alone, again. Just like when I was 12, 13, 18, or 20. I was not alone in it. But it was not talked about. And sometimes, I didn't want to talk about it. But many times I did, and I didn't know who I could talk to. Who could relate? I now know dozens of women who have gone through similar circumstances, but at the time they were not available to me, or I was not available to them.

I began to become curious about the connection between eating disorders and fertility. I had not been able to find many books or articles on the topic, although these issues were showing up with my clients. When the Eating Recovery Center put out a call for proposals for their 2017 conference, I jumped at the opportunity to put together a proposal to speak on this topic. It was warmly received. I was told that this is such a needed discussion, and so I began the chapter of my professional career that began to focus specifically on fertility, eating disorders, and motherhood.

The more I spoke about this, the more I realized that many couples go through what Jeff and I went through. I have worked with numerous clients who have had a similar journey. Let's talk about this more. Let's reduce the shame and find more acceptance. No one chooses to have an eating disorder, and no one chooses to have infertility. If we can band together and create a safe space to talk about uncomfortable things and to help each other heal, it is my hope that we can reduce feelings of isolation and shame related to fertility issues and eating disorders. This is why I am writing this book.

Here you will find the stories of dozens of women who have experienced something related to my experience. Women who are warriors of infertility, who have endured or are still dealing with eating disorders, who are called to connect with their deepest values in a way that they never had done before. These brave women join me to share their narratives so that hopefully the hundreds and thousands of other women around the world who are experiencing similar difficulties and struggles will no longer feel isolated.

Each case study included in this book is a true story. Names and any identifying information have been changed to protect the confidentiality of the participants. The book is divided into several sections: Overview of the Research, which introduces and delves into the current research on these topics; Conception; Pregnancy; Postpartum Attachment and Motherhood; Shame and Perfectionism; and What the Medical Community Needs to Know to Support Clients. The sections that follow the process of pregnancy from conception to postpartum look at two specific population cohorts: women who are in recovery who struggle to get pregnant; and women who have an active eating disorder who intentionally or unintentionally get pregnant. These are their stories from shame to self-acceptance. Included is research already completed on these topics and clinical tools for therapists to use with clients in these populations, as well as questions for therapists to consider to deepen their exploration and understanding of this.

Thank you for being a part of the mission and picking up this book. You may fall under one of the categories that are described in this book, you may know someone who does, or you may be one of the participants who helped me gather my anecdotal research. My hope is that shame and secrecy regarding infertility and eating disorders (two experiences that can tell a person that they are worthless and broken) will be dissolved and healing, acceptance, and connection can begin.

Notes

1. Homepage. (n.d.). Retrieved December 28, 2018, from https://resolve.org/
2. National Center for Health Statistics 2006–2010. (2018, December 19). Retrieved December 28, 2018, from www.cdc.gov/nchs/nsfg/index.htm
3. National Center for Health Statistics 2006–2010. (2018, December 19). Retrieved December 28, 2018, from www.cdc.gov/nchs/nsfg/index.htm
4. Home. (2018). Retrieved December 28, 2018, from https://connect.asrm.org/home?ssopc=1
5. National Women's Health Resource Center. (n.d.). Retrieved December 28, 2018, from https://rarediseases.org/organizations/national-womens-health-resource-center
6. Mercer, W. M. (1997). Infertility as a Covered Benefit. Retrieved December 28, 2018, from https://resolve.org/infertility-101/what-is-infertility/fast-facts/
7. Mercer, W. M. (1997). *Infertility as a covered benefit*. Retrieved December 28, 2018, from https://resolve.org/infertility-101/what-is-infertility/fast-facts/
8. Home. (n.d.). Retrieved December 28, 2018, from https://connect.asrm.org/home?ssopc=1
9. ART Success Rates. (2018, September 11). Retrieved December 28, 2018, from www.cdc.gov/art/artdata/index.html
10. Statistics & Research on Eating Disorders. (2018, September 14). Retrieved December 28, 2018, from www.nationaleatingdisorders.org/statistics-research-eating-disorders
11. DSM-5. (2013). *Diagnostic and statistical manual of mental disorders*. Arlington, VA: American Psychiatric Association.

1 Overview of the Research

Kate Daigle

In this chapter, you'll get a sense of the current research on the topics of fertility, pregnancy, and the postpartum period in relation to eating disorder recovery as well as more thorough descriptions of what eating disorders are. This chapter builds a foundation of understanding of these issues in order to further enrich the case studies, enhance clinical tools that therapists can use with clients, and pose more questions about ethical and comprehensive treatment of eating disorders and infertility. We will go through an overview of the medical, emotional, cognitive, and social complications that having an eating disorder can have on conceiving and producing a healthy child.

Many people with eating disorders or who are in recovery from an eating disorder desire to become pregnant but come across complications and fertility issues. What are the factors that can cause this? And in women with a history of ED and with fertility issues, are we able to tell what is related to an eating disorder and what is not related at all? These questions and more will be further explored.

This book will focus on understanding the lived experience of two populations of women: (1) women who have a sustained eating disorder recovery and who desire to get pregnant but struggle to achieve this; and (2) women who are active in an eating disorder and who get pregnant, either intentionally or unintentionally.

A common underlying theme for both of the populations that I am focusing on is the experience of shame. As I will explain further, there is a high rate of unintended pregnancy in women with current eating disorders, and the decision of how to proceed with the pregnancy can trigger intense self-judgment and fear. Also, in the population of women who strongly desire to have a family and who are in steady ED recovery, unpredicted struggles to conceive can lead the woman to wonder, "Is this my fault?" Concurrently, a sustained eating disorder in early life may cause a woman to choose or need to delay starting a family until she is at "mature maternal age" (35 and over) and fully recovered from her eating disorder. A woman in this age range will risk the chance of fertility challenges whether she has had an ED or not, and possible infertility issues that may arise for a woman in this category can trigger feelings of guilt, shame, and loss as well as the pressure of the "ticking biological clock."

To set us on a solid foundation, let's first get a good understanding of what eating disorders are. According to the *Diagnostic and Statistical Manual of Mental Disorders*, Fifth Edition (DSM-5), "feeding and eating disorders are characterized by a persistent disturbance of eating or eating-related behavior that results in the altered consumption or absorption of food and that significantly impairs physical health or psychosocial functioning."[1] The eating disorders that will be the focus of this book are anorexia nervosa (AN), bulimia nervosa (BN), binge eating disorder (BED), and otherwise specified feeding and eating disorder (OSFED). While the DSM describes several other eating disorder diagnoses such as avoidant/restrictive food intake disorder (ARFID), we will focus primarily on the four major disorders listed above to allow for deeper understanding and exploration.

Also note that the majority of eating disorders do not fit into one specific category (such as the ones listed above) but may be a mix of symptoms or are "subclinical," meaning they do not meet the criteria for a DSM diagnosis but may be equally disruptive to mental and physical health. OSFED, which in prior versions of the DSM was called eating disorder not otherwise specified (EDNOS), captures a large majority of eating disorders that do not fall into the categories of the three main disorders (AN, BN, and BED). We will explore how specific eating disorders affect fertility and health as well as how an ED in general affects this.

Anorexia nervosa is characterized by three essential features: persistent energy intake restriction; intense fear of gaining weight or of becoming fat, or persistent behavior that interferes with weight gain; and a disturbance in self-perceived weight or shape (DSM). There are two subcategories to the diagnosis of anorexia: restricting type and binge/purge type. Those with anorexia maintain a steady weight that is below the normal and natural average weight range for their body by restricting food intake, and they develop medical complications due to this.[2] Atypical anorexia is often overlooked or misdiagnosed, as many people in this category are within normal weight ranges but exhibit the same symptoms of anorexia as listed above. This can lead someone going through this to a feeling of being "invisibilized," or not seen for the severity of their eating disorder. Atypical representations of eating disorders are common across the spectrum of the disorders.

Many of the physical complications of anorexia are due to effects of starvation. In a woman, a major marker of this disease is amenorrhea, or the loss of her period. Primary amenorrhea occurs when a woman age 15 or older never has had her period, and secondary amenorrhea occurs in a woman who has had regular periods but loses her period for a time span of 3 months or more. The loss of menstruation prohibits egg production and shuts down the reproductive system. Hypothalamic amenorrhea, a component of secondary amenorrhea, is common in people with anorexia and occurs when the hypothalamus, which is in the center of the brain and controls reproduction, stops producing gonadotropin-releasing hormone (GnRH). This is the hormone that starts the menstrual cycle, and it can stop it if it does not sense sustainability. One of the factors of this is low body weight, which may or may not be connected to an eating disorder.[3]

When the body is forced into starvation mode, as occurs in anorexia, the brain goes into protection mode. This reaction can be called our "animal brain" or our "caveman brain," as it does not process events mindfully or slowly; it senses danger and potential death, and so it acts on its most primal instinct. It comes from the days of our ancestors, where threats to our survival were plentiful—a neighboring village attacking our village, a bear or mountain lion coming for our young. We needed to be vigilant and on alert at all times.

In this state of "fight, flight or freeze," our bodies feel stressed to preserve as many internal resources as they possibly can. They also recognize that this is not a time suitable for procreation.

When a person is dealing with severe anorexia, the brain can go into this same self-protection and fear mindset. It may sense that death could be imminent, as there is very little or inconsistent fuel coming into the body to sustain it. Thus the brain can shut down "non-essential" organs to preserve what little energy it does have and revert to prepubescent times.

A mature female's brain, when starved, will shut down sex hormones, shrink her ovaries, and eliminate her period until it is deemed "safe" enough to revert to their normal state.[4] Safe in these terms would mean sustained nutrition for an extended period of time. For some women, it can take up to a year of recovery for her to get her period back and her hormones regulated.

Thus, a diagnosis of anorexia nervosa decreases a woman's ability to get pregnant, as her body does not have the resources to offer to the reproductive process during this time of "danger." Even with these factors, women with AN are still getting pregnant—at an alarmingly high rate, which I will expand on in the next chapter. This can understandably pose severe physical and emotional challenges for both mother and baby, as the mother is thrown into a tailspin managing her pregnancy and her eating disorder.

For a woman desiring to have a family, the most important thing she can do is to dedicate herself to full recovery from her eating disorder before trying to conceive. There are severe risks to a pregnancy if a woman is active in AN and is carrying a child; this will be further explored in a future chapter.

Bulimia nervosa has three essential features: recurrent episodes of binge eating, recurrent inappropriate compensatory behaviors to prevent weight gain, and self-evaluation that is unduly influenced by body shape and weight. Binge eating and inappropriate compensatory behaviors must occur at least once per week for 3 months.[5]

Menstrual irregularities are also common in females with bulimia nervosa, though it is not certain whether these disturbances are related to weight fluctuations, nutritional deficiencies, hormonal imbalances, emotional stress, or a combination of these.[6] Bingeing and purging behaviors can flush the body of needed nutrients, cause dehydration, and result in hormone imbalance. People with bulimia are at risk of potassium deficiency from purging, which can lead to irregular heartbeats and cardiac issues. The body is sustained at a high rate of stress during bulimic episodes and can shut down hormone production, most importantly estrogen, which is needed for reproduction.[7] Women in recovery from bulimia can get their hormones back in balance with sustained nutrition and vitamins and cessation of eating disorder behaviors. There are significant risks to a pregnancy if a woman is active in BN while she is carrying a child. This will be further explored in a subsequent chapter.

Binge eating disorder is the most common of the classified eating disorders, and it just recently received official diagnostic criteria in the most recent version of the DSM-5 in 2013. It has a more equal male-to-female gender ratio, with about 40% of those with BED being male. Of those with anorexia, about 25% are males and of those with bulimia, about 25% are males.[8]

The essential feature of binge eating disorder is recurrent episodes of binge eating that must occur, on average, at least once per week for 3 months. Binge eating is defined as feeling out of control while eating, and eating an amount of food in a discrete period of time that is more than most people would eat in a similar period of time under similar circumstances.[9] Many people with BED are overweight, but a significant amount are in a normal weight range and the disorder can go undetected in this group of people who may also feel invisibilized, or not seen. With the amount of weight stigma in our society today, people in larger bodies may be told to "just lose weight" or go on a diet in order to be healthy by their medical provider, which at the very least may make them feel unheard and could put them at risk for an eating disorder to develop or go unassessed. Menstrual irregularities are also common in BED, especially if a woman is overweight or obese. Obesity in women can result in high levels of androgens, or male hormones, which can cause abnormal menstrual cycles and block ovulation.[10]

If a woman in a larger body who struggles with BED goes to her doctor to try to understand why she is having menstrual irregularities, she is most likely going to be told to lose weight, with doctors often assuming it must be polycystic ovary syndrome (PCOS). Women who are in smaller bodies who also struggle with BED are more likely to be asked many questions about their medical history and have their doctor investigate multiple possibilities for the disruption. A Health at Every Size (HAES™)[11] approach works to bring back menstrual function in any size of woman and focuses on her overall mental and physical health, not just the number on the scale.[12] This will be explored further in Chapter 7.

I want to add here that there is also other specified feeding or eating disorder (OSFED), which describes an eating disturbance that may carry factors of any of the above described disorders but does not fit the clinical standards for diagnosis. These eating disturbances can be equally damaging to a woman's physical and emotional wellness and risk going undetected or not seen as "true eating disorders."

So How Do Eating Disorders Affect Fertility?

Eating disorders affect many women at a childbearing age. Research shows that eating disorders affect 5.2%–6.5% of young females, but they often go undetected in health care and the number could be even higher.[13] This may be due to an atypical eating disorder not being recognized for what it is or hesitancy on the part of the client to admit she has a disorder. Contrary to popular belief, many women with eating disorders are getting pregnant despite significant menstrual irregularities, and it is reported that an increasing number of women with anorexia and bulimia are reporting unintended pregnancies. While most women with anorexia halt all egg production due to restriction, some women have intermittent egg production, meaning they release an egg intermittently, not each month.[14] Women may not think they can get pregnant when they have anorexia and not use contraception, but they can be mistaken.

In women with current eating disorders, there is an elevated risk of pregnancy complications and adverse effects to both mother and child.[15] In recent studies, there were increased rates of miscarriages and induced abortions in the prenatal period for both AN and BN. Binge eating disorder is often (but not always) associated with a higher than average body mass index (BMI), which itself has a higher rate of miscarriage and increased risk of stillbirth. In Linna's study, it was found that women with a lifetime eating disorder (meaning spanning almost their entire life) more commonly were childless than women without an ED.[16] This may be due to complications in conceiving and carrying a baby to term, that they delayed trying to start a family due to the presence of an ED or being in treatment, or that they felt they could not be a good parent or were not willing to give up their ED to care for a child.

In women with AN, pregnancy rates were less than half of the rates of the control group; induced abortions were most common in women with lifetime BN, and miscarriages were most common in women with lifetime BED. Miscarriages were surprisingly frequent in BED, as women with BED had a miscarriage in almost half of their pregnancies.[17] This will be further explored in Chapter 2 on conception.

There are also impulsive personality traits at play in clients with BN (and some with AN, as a woman may perceive that she is not ovulating) and with a mixture of AN/BN, which can lead to risky behavior and higher rates of unplanned pregnancies. This might mean unprotected sexual activity and irrational thinking patterns about what the consequences might be.

There is insufficient research into the intersection of EDs and fertility issues, especially in populations that do not fit into a specific ED diagnosis or that are subclinical. In what has been researched, it has been found that disturbed menses is common criteria for women with AN, and even can persist in up to 30% in women who have recovered from AN.[18] However, a recent study found a fairly high incidence of women coming to fertility treatment centers who meet criteria for an ED, which is 16%–20%. The number of births in women with AN has been shown to be one-third of the expected rate. Also, of the women with AN, 40% reported that their pregnancy was unintentional.

Difficulty bonding with the baby in the womb, which could be a result of an eating disorder or other issues, has been shown to predict poor postpartum attachment between mother and child.[19] This can have long-term consequences for the mother-child relationship and may be a result of the mother's own unhealthy attachment pattern from her childhood that she has not repaired. A recent study found that more than 90% of women with a history of EDs reported problems regarding their adjustment at 3 months postpartum, compared with 13% of women who had not had an eating disorder.[20]

In a groundbreaking study by Easter, it was found that across all eating disorder types (AN, BN, and BED), negative impressions about discovering their pregnancy were more common than in the general population. Women with lifetime AN reported their pregnancy as a "personal sacrifice," having to battle between the eating disorder identity and the maternal identity. Fear of losing their eating disorder was strong. Weight gain, which is healthy and inevitable in pregnancy, also challenged the coping ability of many women with AN and made them resentful of their growing bodies.[21]

Easter also found that women in this study had a complex relationship with prenatal bonding, which means bonding with the child while it is in the womb. Prenatal bonding may be indicative of postpartum attachment, as noted earlier, and many women do reduce ED symptoms and focus on bonding with their unborn child instead of the ED. For these women, nurturing their bodies because it is holding and growing a child is easier and holds a bigger purpose than nurturing their bodies for their own health.

Unfortunately there is a high rate of ED relapse in the postpartum period of up to 60%–70%, and women with a history of EDs are also at increased risk of developing postpartum depression or anxiety,[22] which will be explored further in Chapter 4.

Having a child is one of the most significant life transitions a woman can encounter. It is shown that in studies across different countries, 10%–20% of women report experiencing an episode of depression in the first few months after giving birth. From 7% to 15% of women report having an episode of depression in late pregnancy. Multiple studies have confirmed a link between previous depressive disorders, increasing the risk of these types of disorders resurfacing in the perinatal period (the weeks immediately before and after birth).[23]

It has been found that eating disorders have a high rate of comorbidity with major depressive disorder and anxiety disorders. There is much less known about the connection and presence of these disorders in women who are pregnant or in the postpartum period and who have had an eating disorder.

How Does Male Infertility Factor In?

According to research, infertility is one-third related to the female partner, one-third is attributed to the male partner, and one-third is unexplained.[24] We have explored some of the physical effects that an eating disorder has on a woman's fertility, but not much is written about the impact of an eating disorder on a man's fertility.

In our culture, weight stigma is prevalent, and medical professionals have long subscribed to the idea that fertility in both men and women is directly related to serum leptin levels. Leptin is a fat-tissue-based hormone that manages the function of reproductive hormones and is also responsible for bone and blood formation, metabolism, appetite, and normal neuropeptide function.[25] However, this prejudicial viewpoint is not weight inclusive and highlights that weight and "health" have been erroneously linked for many years. New data has shown that the linkage between pure body weight and certain outcomes are less clear and many diverse factors may contribute to fertility complications.

As two-thirds of fertility patients (male and female) who are actively restricting are in the average BMI range (18.5–25), many of these patients do not self-report their ED symptoms to their doctor and may not be assessed for these behaviors.[26]

For many women struggling to get pregnant, a primary issue they are experiencing is amenorrhea or oligomenorrhea (absence of or irregular menstrual cycle, respectively). Anovular infertility is a state in which a menstrual cycle happens but no egg has been released.

> Anovular infertility is common in women who have only partially recovered [from eating disorders]. Terming this hypothalamic anovulation is misleading and dangerous, as it leads to medical intervention to induce pregnancy. This is unwise, as the pregnancies of such women are known to have more complications, result in more premature births, and to be associated with poor Apgar scores[27]* and underweight neonates.[28]

Women may not bring up to their doctor having a current eating disorder if they are experiencing anovular infertility due to stigma around mental health, and their OB-GYN will most likely not assess for eating disorders at this time.

For men, infertility and eating disorders both carry a heavy sense of shame and stigma, even more so than for women where these issues are more discussed and understood. Eating disorders in men may cause poor fertility health in the form of low testosterone levels, which are the male reproductive hormones (estrogen in women). Men in Western society are held to standards that are also unattainable: to be "masculine" and not show any strong emotion (except perhaps anger), especially if it is a vulnerable one. Physically they are expected to be muscular (but not too muscular), or thin and fit. Restriction or excessive exercise are utilized by men to try to control their appearance to attract partners and to be more accepted by our culture.[29]

When the idea of infertility is brought to mind, it is not normally a man that one might think of, though it occurs as frequently in men as it does in women. Men might struggle with feeling emasculated or unable to live up to their responsibility as a "man" and may feel guilt, shame, anger, and other complex emotions. Much as when a woman feels shame at not meeting expectations to be a mother if she struggles with infertility, men may feel similar shame but not feel as comfortable to talk about it. Hence, many men do not bring up these issues with their doctor, friends, partners, or support system.

A recent study found that only 41% of OB/GYN physicians considered a urological evaluation of the male partner, and only 24% would routinely refer the male partner to a urologist before ordering a semen analysis. Male infertility can be caused by structural abnormalities, sperm production disorders, ejaculatory disorders, and immunologic disorders, among other things.[30]

The direct link between eating disorders and fertility in males warrants further research, and currently fertility doctors have been treating anorexia in men with prescribing weight restoration and exercise cessation if they are excessively exercising. Counseling is recommended to focus on the sources and maintaining factors of their eating disorder, although willingness to see a therapist for this issue may be lessened due to stigma. In the past decade or so, a new intervention has been administered by doctors: treating men with eating disorders (specifically anorexia) with transdermal (through the skin), oral, or injected testosterone. Many patients, both male and female, are treated with hormones and medication to improve fertility without informed and effective assessment of overall mental and physical wellness, including eating disorders.

There are risks to administering pharmaceuticals to a patient without treating the underlying causes, which, when treated successfully, can help improve fertility naturally. This is a risk for both male and female fertility patients.

Ryan, 33, and his wife Katie, 31, have been married for 3 years and have been ready to start a family for the past year. In getting their prenatal checkups with their doctor, Ryan was told that his testosterone levels were very low, and this might be part of the reason that they have not yet conceived. Ryan was an elite runner in college, competing in track and field on a scholarship and becoming very connected to his athlete identity. He learned that the faster he ran, the more accolades he got and the higher his self-esteem rose. To run faster, he began cutting calories and became excessively rigid about and hyperfocused on his diet. No one knew the extent of his exercise habits and the degree to how out of control he began to feel about his relationship to food. He felt ashamed that it had "gotten to this point," but he did not know how to get himself out of the hole he was in. He was able to continue and make great times competing despite feeling much weaker physically, and after college he went on to do triathlons and marathons regularly.

When he met Katie, he opened up to her about the toll that his exercise and diet habits had on him, and that he felt like he "couldn't cut back and felt like he had to keep pushing his training," running up to eight miles a day. She was able to help him realize that the life they were building together was more important than his disorder and encouraged him to get counseling, which he did. Ryan reports that he has had a "pretty normal" relationship with food and has cut back to running twice a week for the past 4 years. He didn't think that his past disorder could affect his fertility, and

> now that he knows that his hormones were so disrupted by years of physical abuse to my body, I feel so much shame. I didn't want to tell my doctor about my past, it's too hard. Katie convinced me to open up to my doctor about it and I'm trying to make sure I'm healthy overall right now to further our chances of getting pregnant. No one talks about male infertility, and no one talks about men with eating disorders. It just isn't a "thing" you talk about, I guess.

Ryan and Katie are waiting on trying any fertility treatments until Ryan improves his diet and balances out his stress management. His doctor recommends giving him testosterone injections, but Ryan wants to try to first improve his hormonal balance naturally.

With knowledge of how high the relapse rate of an eating disorder can be in new parenthood for both women and men, what are the risks to treating fertility patients without a full assessment of ED and mental health? For someone who is active in an ED, their mental and physical stability are decompensated, and going through fertility treatments without ensuring a solid foundation of recovery may put the parent and, ultimately, the child in a position of unstable ground. This may contribute to poor parent-child attachment while the child is in the womb and postpartum. Medical doctors are strongly encouraged to be assessing for mental health issues, such as eating disorders, before administering any type of fertility treatment.

Attachment

Attachment, which means the parent's ability to attune to their child's needs and bond with their child in the postpartum period, is an area of clinical interest and significance among women with an active or past ED. In a 2016 study performed by Sadeh-Sharvit et al., it was found that a maternal eating disorder increased the risk of feeding or eating problems in young children as well as binge, emotional, or restrictive eating in their children as they grow older.[31] There is some preliminary research that suggests that maternal EDs affect their child's general development; for example, a mother may feel her child is too needy, has a negative temperament, and displays less happiness than the child of a mother with no ED history. Mother-child bonding in women with a history of ED is an area that warrants much more research.

Analysis of research that has been completed on this topic shows that in feeding interactions between a mother with an ED and her child there is greater conflict, more maternal controlling behaviors, and less positive emotion towards her child during mealtimes compared to women with no ED. The mother's own concern with her eating habits and weight was translated into an overattentiveness in her child's eating habits and weight and resulted in less pleasant eating environments and overall bonding with her child. It has been found, however, that these differences were not replicated in women who had fully recovered from their ED.[32]

Sadeh-Sharvit's study is unique in that it begins to explore the connection between mothers with EDs and the way their emotions and ED symptomology affects bonding with their child in a feeding environment. There is a need for more research on how a mother's ED might impact the child's development more fully in other areas of his/her life. One hypothesis about this is that the mother may have impairment of emotional availability. Emotional availability is a theory that emphasizes the dyadic nature of the mother-child interaction and how this influences the child's overall well-being. Maternal mental disorders are associated with a decreased capacity for the mother to accurately be able to attune and respond to their child's needs (inhibiting their capacity to be emotionally available).[33] This has, however, not yet been systematically studied among mothers with EDs and their children.

Looking further into the concept of emotional availability gives us more insight into the factors that impact the mother-child relationship. Mothers with a lifetime ED are known to have greater anxiety, cognitive inflexibility and harm avoidance, and lower self-efficacy. In the feeding arena, mother-child interactions are impacted by significant controlling behaviors in this population. If a mother is preoccupied with her own anxiety, depression, or ED symptoms, she may not be as emotionally available to her child. In the only two studies completed on playtime dynamics in this population, one found more intrusiveness in mothers with EDs but no fewer positive expressed emotions, and one found in mothers who were fully recovered no decrease in sensitivity.[34] Mothers with a lifetime ED may translate their inner world (higher risk avoidance, control, rigidity) to their parenting style.

In Sadeh-Sharvit's current study, emotional availability of a mother with an ED towards her child was measured in feeding environments as well as outside of eating.

Their findings suggest that mothers with lifetime EDs and their toddlers displayed less adaptive emotional responsiveness than mothers who had recovered. Mothers with EDs tended to view their children more negatively, which then was translated to their child's tendency to view the world that way too. This also can put the children at risk for developing an ED themselves, adopting coping styles that they perceive as familiar.

Another study looked at the impact of women who currently have BN on their attachment to their children. They found that women with active BN were overly preoccupied with their own as well as their child's weight and attempted to slim down their infants as early as the first postnatal year. In addition, these mothers were more concerned with their daughters' weight than their sons'. These mothers also had abnormal feeding practices such as feeding their infants on a less regular basis and using food for non-nutritive purposes (reward, expressing love). During mealtimes, high rates of anxiety were common. Mothers underfed their children or have difficulty preparing meals to avoid being triggered to go into their own binge cycle.[35] This will be explored in more depth in Chapter 4.

There are many risks to fertility and motherhood when a mother has a current or recent eating disorder. Conversely, when a woman is fully recovered, there is no medical reason she should have any additional complications to her fertility than a woman who has never had an ED; however, she may experience shame or guilt if she encounters infertility during her journey to becoming a parent. This topic is comprehensive, and is an umbrella under which emotional, social, mental, and physical health factors of both mother and child are affected and development of the baby and the mother-child bond may be impacted by the presence of an ED. This book will focus on these topics, interviews with women on different phases of this journey will be included, and tools and discussion will be provided to help explore the roots of this shame and transition it to self-acceptance.

So much is hidden and unspoken in regard to both fertility issues and eating disorders. They are called "invisible struggles," which fester and fuel underneath the surface. It is my hope that this book will shed a light on the lived experiences of women, including myself, who have gone through or are currently experiencing these challenges and allow them to be seen and heard as a group who share these struggles but are not defined by them.

Notes

1. DSM-5. (2013). *Diagnostic and statistical manual of mental disorders: DSM-5*. Arlington, VA: American Psychiatric Association.
2. DSM-5. (2013). *Diagnostic and statistical manual of mental disorders: DSM-5*. Arlington, VA: American Psychiatric Association.

3. What causes amenorrhea? (n.d.). Retrieved December 28, 2018, from www.nichd.nih.gov/health/topics/amenorrhea/conditioninfo/causes
4. Kimmel, M., Ferguson, E., Zerwas, S., Bulik, C., & Meltzer-Brody, S. (2015). Obstetric and gynecologic problems associated with eating disorders. *International Journal of Eating Disorders*, *49*(3), 260–275. https://doi.org/10.1002/eat.22483
5. DSM-5. (2013). *Diagnostic and statistical manual of mental disorders: DSM-5*. Arlington, VA: American Psychiatric Association.
6. DSM-5. (2013). *Diagnostic and statistical manual of mental disorders: DSM-5*. Arlington, VA: American Psychiatric Association.
7. DSM-5. (2013). *Diagnostic and statistical manual of mental disorders: DSM-5*. Arlington, VA: American Psychiatric Association.
8. Statistics & Research on Eating Disorders. (2018, September 14). Retrieved December 28, 2018, from www.nationaleatingdisorders.org/statistics-research-eating-disorders
9. DSM-5. (2013). *Diagnostic and statistical manual of mental disorders: DSM-5*. Arlington, VA: American Psychiatric Association.
10. Pasquali, R. (2006). Obesity and androgens: Facts and perspectives. *Fertility and Sterility*, *85*(5), 1319–1340. https://doi.org/10.1016/j.fertnstert.2005.10.054
11. Health At Every Size and HAES are registered trademarks of the Association for Size Diversity and Health and used with permission.
12. Health at Every Size®. (n.d.). Retrieved December 28, 2018, from https://haescommunity.com/
13. Linna, M.S., Raevuori, A., Haukka, J., Suvisaari, J.M., Suokas, J.T., & Gissler, M. (2013). Reproductive health outcomes in eating disorders. *International Journal of Eating Disorders*, *46*(8), 826–833. https://doi.org/10.1002/eat.22179
14. Bulik, C.M., Hoffman, E.R., Holle, A.V., Torgersen, L., Stoltenberg, C., & Reichborn-Kjennerud, T. (2010). Unplanned pregnancy in women with anorexia nervosa. *Obstetrics & Gynecology*, *116*(5), 1136–1140. https://doi.org/10.1097/aog.0b013e3181f7efdc
15. Linna, M.S., Raevuori, A., Haukka, J., Suvisaari, J.M., Suokas, J.T., & Gissler, M. (2013). Reproductive health outcomes in eating disorders. *International Journal of Eating Disorders*, *46*(8), 826–833. https://doi.org/10.1002/eat.22179
16. Linna, M.S., Raevuori, A., Haukka, J., Suvisaari, J.M., Suokas, J.T., & Gissler, M. (2013). Reproductive health outcomes in eating disorders. *International Journal of Eating Disorders*, *46*(8), 826–833. https://doi.org/10.1002/eat.22179
17. Linna, M.S., Raevuori, A., Haukka, J., Suvisaari, J.M., Suokas, J.T., & Gissler, M. (2013). Reproductive health outcomes in eating disorders. *International Journal of Eating Disorders*, *46*(8), 826–833. https://doi.org/10.1002/eat.22179
18. Easter, A., Treasure, J., & Micali, N. (2011). Fertility and prenatal attitudes towards pregnancy in women with eating disorders: Results from the Avon longitudinal study of parents and children. *BJOG: An International Journal of Obstetrics & Gynaecology*, *118*(12), 1491–1498. https://doi.org/10.1111/j.1471-0528.2011.03077.x
19. Fogarty, S., Elmir, R., Hay, P., & Schmied, V. (2018). The experience of women with an eating disorder in the perinatal period: A meta-ethnographic study. *BMC Pregnancy and Childbirth*, *18*(1). https://doi.org/10.1186/s12884-018-1762-9
20. Easter, A., Treasure, J., & Micali, N. (2011). Fertility and prenatal attitudes towards pregnancy in women with eating disorders: Results from the Avon Longitudinal Study of Parents and Children. *BJOG: An International Journal of Obstetrics & Gynaecology*, *118*(12), 1491–1498. https://doi.org/10.1111/j.1471-0528.2011.03077.x

21. Easter, A., Treasure, J., & Micali, N. (2011). Fertility and prenatal attitudes towards pregnancy in women with eating disorders: Results from the Avon longitudinal study of parents and children. *BJOG: An International Journal of Obstetrics & Gynaecology*, *118*(12), 1491–1498. https://doi.org/10.1111/j.1471-0528.2011.03077.x
22. Micali, N., Simonoff, E., & Treasure, J. (2011). Pregnancy and post-partum depression and anxiety in a longitudinal general population cohort: The effect of eating disorders and past depression. *Journal of Affective Disorders*, *131*(1–3), 150–157. https://doi.org/10.1016/j.jad.2010.09.034
23. Micali, N., Simonoff, E., & Treasure, J. (2011). Pregnancy and post-partum depression and anxiety in a longitudinal general population cohort: The effect of eating disorders and past depression. *Journal of Affective Disorders*, *131*(1–3), 150–157. https://doi.org/10.1016/j.jad.2010.09.034
24. HOME. (n.d.). Retrieved December 28, 2018, from https://connect.asrm.org/home?ssopc=1
25. Olwyn, G. (2011, November 11). *Reproductive health I: Fertility & pregnancy*. Retrieved December 30, 2018, from https://edinstitute.org/paper/2011/11/11/reproductive-health-i-fertility-pregnancy
26. Olwyn, G. (2011, November 11). *Reproductive health I: Fertility & pregnancy*. Retrieved December 30, 2018, from https://edinstitute.org/paper/2011/11/11/reproductive-health-i-fertility-pregnancy
27. Apgar scores: activity (and muscle tone), pulse (heart rate), grimace (reflex irritability), appearance (skin coloration) and respiration (breathing rate and effort to breathe). These are tests that are done for your newborn to assess whether there is an immediate need for further medical care. The scale is 0 to 2, with 2 being the best.
28. D. Gaskill, & Sanders, F. (Eds.). (2000). *The encultured body: Policy implications for healthy body image and disordered eating behaviours*. Brisbane: Queensland University of Technology, p. 81.
29. Mccabe, M. P., & Ricciardelli, L. A. (2004). Body image dissatisfaction among males across the lifespan. *Journal of Psychosomatic Research*, *56*(6), 675–685. doi:10.1016/s0022-3999(03)00129-6
30. Olwyn, G. (2011, November 11). *Reproductive health I: Fertility & pregnancy*. Retrieved December 30, 2018, from https://edinstitute.org/paper/2011/11/11/reproductive-health-i-fertility-pregnancy
31. Sadeh-Sharvit, S., Levy-Shiff, R., Arnow, K.D., & Lock, J.D. (2016). The interactions of mothers with eating disorders with their toddlers: Identifying broader risk factors. *Attachment & Human Development*, *18*(4), 418–428. https://doi.org/10.1080/14616734.2016.1164201
32. Sadeh-Sharvit, S., Levy-Shiff, R., Arnow, K.D., & Lock, J.D. (2016). The interactions of mothers with eating disorders with their toddlers: Identifying broader risk factors. *Attachment & Human Development*, *18*(4), 418–428. https://doi.org/10.1080/14616734.2016.1164201
33. Sadeh-Sharvit, S., Levy-Shiff, R., Arnow, K.D., & Lock, J.D. (2016). The interactions of mothers with eating disorders with their toddlers: Identifying broader risk factors. *Attachment & Human Development*, *18*(4), 418–428. https://doi.org/10.1080/14616734.2016.1164201
34. Lai, B.P., & Tang, C.S. (2008). The negative impact of maternal bulimic symptoms on parenting behavior. *Journal of Psychosomatic Research*, *65*(2), 181–189. https://doi.org/10.1016/j.jpsychores.2008.04.003
35. Lai, B.P., & Tang, C.S. (2008). The negative impact of maternal bulimic symptoms on parenting behavior. *Journal of Psychosomatic Research*, *65*(2), 181–189. https://doi.org/10.1016/j.jpsychores.2008.04.003

2 Conception

> Perhaps strength doesn't reside in having never been broken but in the courage required to grow strong in the broken places.
>
> —Anonymous

The topic of fertility and having children can be complex for women with an eating disorder history, and it can evoke a variety of reactions. We are focusing on two populations: women who have recovered from an ED and desire to get pregnant, and women who have an active eating disorder and get pregnant either intentionally or unintentionally. This path can be paved with fear, shame, excitement, loss, and many other emotions for women in both of these groups.

What does recovery even mean? And what is the difference between recovering and recovered? There are many ideas and opinions about this, but I find myself to align quite solidly with the definition posed by Carolyn Costin, an author and therapist who has recovered from an eating disorder:

> Being recovered to me is when the person can accept his or her natural body size and shape and no longer has a self-destructive or unnatural relationship with food or exercise. When you are recovered, food and weight take a proper perspective in your life and what you weigh is not more important than who you are; in fact, actual numbers are of little or no importance at all. When recovered, you will not compromise your health or betray your soul to look a certain way, wear a certain size or reach a certain number on a scale. When recovered, you do not use eating disorder behaviors to deal with, distract from, or cope with other problems.[1]

In my research and while interviewing dozens of women, I came across many who used the words "recovered" and "in recovery" to describe where they are in their process, and who also had difficulty getting pregnant or sustaining a pregnancy. I also would put myself in this group. I begin to wonder—why? Is there a connection between an ED history and fertility issues? Others said: "I am in recovery, meaning abstaining from behaviors and not allowing ED to control my life. I don't use the term 'recovered' due to the biological factors that cannot be eradicated" and "I don't know at what point I would have considered myself 'recovered'—it's not an on/off switch. It's a process of changing the way you allow yourself to see your body and relationship to nutrition and food."

Whether it is a state of being that one achieves or a gradation of letting go of behaviors and thoughts, being "in recovery" is unique for each person, as is their story, biological components, and personality traits.

Recovery is a nonlinear process, and people in recovery often follow the stages of change process, sometimes looping through it more than once. Getting an understanding of the stages of change process posited by the transtheoretical model and applied to eating disorder recovery helps shed light on factors that influence a woman's readiness to focus on recovery if she is trying to conceive, if she is pregnant, or if she is a new mother.

There are five stages in the recovery process: pre-contemplation, contemplation, preparation, action, and maintenance. Pre-contemplation is qualified by a person not believing they have a problem, while family members and loved ones may see strong symptoms that they are struggling. Contemplation is described as a person being willing to admit that they have a problem and are open to receiving help, even if their fear is very strong. Preparation occurs when a person is ready to make a change but are uncertain how to do it. Their fear may be a little less than their drive to feel better, and they practice coping skills such as assertiveness and boundary setting. The action stage occurs when a person fully invests themselves in the recovery process and takes steps toward recovering from their eating disorder, including changing eating behaviors, and are open to receiving new input. Finally, the maintenance stages consists of maintaining the changes made in recovery, including thought patterns, behaviors, interactions in relationships, self-care, and more. They are in the action stage for 6 months or longer and are actively working to prevent relapse.[2]

Major life events such as getting in a new relationship/getting married, breaking up with a partner/divorce, moving, and having a child are risky situations for those in recovery, especially if they have been in recovery for less than a year. Research shows that recovery can take up to seven years for full cessation of ED and related behaviors and thoughts.[3] A woman who gets pregnant and has a child may revert to old patterns in the contemplation or preparation stage and need to revisit the stages of change process while integrating her new life stage.

Women in Recovery Who Desire to Get Pregnant

For many women who have struggled with an eating disorder, wanting to have a family one day is an incredibly strong value that motivates them to dedicate themselves to recovery. This is especially true for women who are in the stage of life that involves life planning, partner searching, and looking for meaning, usually around the mid- to late twenties.

As the majority of eating disorders begin in the teenage years, it is possible that a woman may have struggled for up to a decade (or more) before choosing to recover fully. Research says that as many as 75%–80% of women will go on to conceive after being successfully treated for an eating disorder and that there is no reason her ED history should affect fertility if she is in sustained physical and emotional recovery. This is to say that there can be medical and emotional factors that can complicate the conception process, but that those are independent of ED factors in sustained recovery.[4]

What happens, though, if one of the underlying values for committing to recovery is one's desire to have a family, and then they struggle to achieve this? They might be unable to conceive or to carry a pregnancy to term. Doctors say there "should" be no ED-related reason for this. But how does this really feel? For me, it was a mixture of feeling shame, fear, and pain and a reconnaissance of some old negative self-beliefs: you're broken; it's your fault.

I had not had those particular thoughts for over a decade, yet they crept back in as if they had never left. I shudder to think of the power of an eating disorder on someone's emotional and mental state; while one can be in full recovery, I believe that the eating disorder is perpetually "in wait" to come back and take over again at any moment of weakness. Someone in recovery can be particularly vulnerable during times of transition or stress where there are unknown or out-of-control factors. Personally, my struggle to get pregnant was the single hardest and most painful experience of my life next to recovering from my ED when I was in my early twenties. I realize that in times of feeling out of control, my old ED voice can attempt to creep back and "help" me to cope.

I have since realized that I was not (and am not) alone—although this was not spoken openly when I needed to hear it most. I heard similar stories from women I met during my writing process.

Nora, 39, has been recovered from anorexia for 10 years, after a 22-year battle with the eating disorder that was triggered by a traumatic childhood. She now works as a therapist helping others who struggle with eating disorders and trauma. She states "I have always wanted to be a mom" and utilized this value as a driving force in her recovery process, which took her to four different treatment centers and numerous therapists and dietitians before she finally found true recovery. Due to the severity of her ED, Nora was not able to focus on getting married and starting a family until she was in her mid-thirties. She met her husband, Joe, when she was 37, and they knew they wanted to start a family together. After trying to get pregnant for several months and not succeeding, they met with a fertility doctor. Nora was open with this doctor about her ED past and the doctor took this into account with his recommendations to her. They tried an egg retrieval, which did not gather as many viable eggs as they Nora and Joe had hoped. She was told her egg quality was poor. They then tried to create embryos, but none of them proceeded to the blastocyst phase. Nora felt shame and guilt. She was angry at the world, at her body, at herself, at her husband, at her past ED, at anything she could project her pain onto. Despite this intense struggle, Nora and Joe got closer and stronger as a couple.

Nora and Joe then proceeded to prepare for intrauterine insemination (IUI), which is a fertility treatment that involves placing sperm inside a woman's uterus to facilitate fertilization. The medication that she was prescribed to help her body ovulate and prepare for pregnancy caused her to lose weight. Her past ED voice was triggered to resurface and "congratulate" her for losing this weight, even though that was the exact opposite thing that Nora needed and wanted to do for her health. Nora's IUI failed and she was devastated once again.

They began to prepare for IVF, which was their doctor's recommendation for best chances of getting pregnant at this point. Nora's doctor recommended that she drastically reduce her exercise and to focus on gaining at least five pounds. Nora had never heard these words from a trusting, supportive source before, and her ED voice was very afraid of this. She needed to weigh herself several times a week now, this time for the purpose of health, not hurting herself as her ED had done in her past. She and her husband have undergone three rounds of egg retrievals and embryo formation and in that course, Nora gained 10 pounds under her doctor's advice. The process was successful: they now have two girl embryos and will do one more round. They will do implantation and hope to be pregnant at the end of 2018. She feels hopeful and excited, with a twinge of nervousness and fear that it might still not work after all they have been through. She states:

> I think my eating disorder took many years from me and delayed my time to get pregnant. However, I am thankful that I waited, as I would never want my child to see me active in an eating disorder. The years of struggling with anorexia probably had an effect on my fertility, but this is something I have had to work through in order to forgive myself.

According to a study published by the journal *Reproductive BioMedicine Online*, over one million couples worldwide go through fertility treatments every year to try to have a child.[5] Upwards of one-third of these couples are told that they have "unexplained" or idiopathic infertility, which translates to the doctors not seeming to be able to find anything wrong with the male's sperm or the female's fallopian tubes or uterus. There are studies now finding out more of the causes of unexplained infertility, but for many of these couples there is still no explanation even after dozens of tests and thousands of dollars spent trying to understand why they cannot conceive. This is devastating for so many of these couples.

Felicia, 33, and her husband Mark have been trying to conceive a child for 3 years. She struggled with anorexia beginning in her sophomore year of high school all through college. She received outpatient therapy and intensive outpatient treatment and was hospitalized several times. She began to recover at the end of her senior year of college and has not displayed any ED behaviors or struggled with the ED impacting her life since that time. She now says, "I am starting to question if the narrative of 'recovered' works for me" (due to her recent challenges with getting pregnant).

> I have been trying to conceive for the past 3.5 years. I have never been pregnant. I have tried medication (Clomid cycles), and have had two failed IUI's and I have undergone three rounds of IVF. It was found that my egg quality was poor and we have gone through two failed embryo transfers. My fertility is diagnosed as "unexplained." However, during my eating disorder, I lost my period for several years. I have a distinct memory of a therapist asking, "Do you want to have kids ever, or do you want to be skinny?" I said I wanted to be skinny. Now I carry a lot of guilt about that. I know the research is inconclusive about long-term amenorrhea and its connection to infertility, but I *firmly* believe that a decade of living well below my set point has had a negative effect on my infertility. I have now paused all fertility treatments for the foreseeable future. I fear that I may be a hopeless case.

She continues:

> I carry shame from the question posed to me years ago by my old therapist. I have had fearful thoughts of my infertility being fate-intervening because perhaps I would pass an eating disorder to my child, would make an unfit mother, or that pregnancy would cause a relapse for me. I sought out a support group, but there are none in my area. Currently I am searching for a therapist who specializes in infertility but this has also been a struggle. I would say that leaning on my husband and family members has been the most helpful thus far.

Felicia is now a psychologist, and although she doesn't work with people with eating disorders or fertility issues, she feels that her past and current struggles have influenced her to want to help others who suffer from mental and physical health issues.

The desire to have something in one's control is often a maintaining factor of an eating disorder. The experience of infertility is the utmost definition of loss of control. Renée, 32, underwent an experience similar to Felicia's. She is soon to begin her first (and only) embryo transfer; her egg retrieval produced nine eggs, which was a wonderful result. After analyzing the eggs, however, the doctors found that the quality was poor and only two viable embryos grew, both of lower quality. While awaiting the embryo transfer and injecting herself with a plethora of hormones such as estrogen and progesterone, Renée found herself resorting to old restricting and controlling behaviors to cope with the stress of the situation and the not-knowing. She felt anxious and distressed when her house was not clean, something that would have never bothered her before. She felt symptoms of panic when things did not go as she expected at work, with her husband, with their dog. She had been eating a more diverse and less rigid diet for the past 6 months to try to get her body healthy enough to get pregnant and carry a child. The news of the poor egg quality sent her back into old habits with eating and exercise—not as severe as a couple of years earlier, but serving as another way to attempt a form of control.

For women such as Felicia and Renée and their partners, who may be the "silent sufferers" in infertility, counseling can be effective in reducing shame and bringing compassion and connection to the couple.

Clinical Tools for Working With Individuals or Couples Going Through Infertility

Treasure Map of Infertility Journey

Create a treasure map of the infertility journey; other journeys may converge with this one—kids from previous relationship, ED recovery, learning about infertility before relationship, and so forth. What mountains they have climbed, cliffs they've fallen off of, rivers they've waded across, places they have rested, stormy seas, hidden treasures.[6]

Weaving a Nest: Can Be Done in Group Setting, Couples, or Individually

The individual/group weaves a "nest" of yarn together as they share difficult feelings. Each person weaves their yarn as they talk, and then they pass it on to the next person. Once the nest is complete, *so* many things can be done with it. They can write on strips of paper the grief and shame they feel regarding the infertility, or any emotions or intentions they want to get out. The nest can be kept in the therapist's office or elsewhere as a resource for healing and processing.[7]

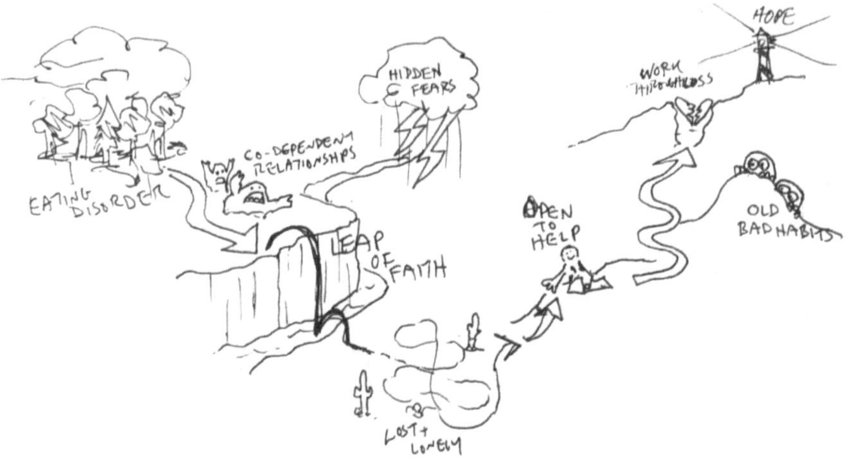

Figure 2.1 An example of a treasure map highlighting a woman's infertility and eating disorder journey

Shame Container

Creating a "shame container" can sometimes help access and heal shame if it is viewed and processed in a less overwhelming setting. The therapist provides small boxes (matchboxes, tea containers, shoe boxes, etc.) and asks the client to decorate the outside of the box with collage or drawing/painting imagery representing how they show their shame (or hide it away) to the outside world. Then on the inside they can use imagery and collage, as well as writing, objects, photographs, and so forth to depict what their shame feels like inside.[8]

Building on Mindfulness and Guided Imagery

Guide client to a state of mindfulness through guided imagery or journaling that gently and empathetically puts them in touch with their shame. Then guide them to locate/describe/image what this shame experience feels like (and do it, again, in a way that builds empathy). Then guide them to make the connection with how their eating disorder experiences (or tries to avoid experiencing) this shame through food behaviors and their body—in a deep kind of way, for example, "there is something wrong and defective with me/my body" and "if I restrict it/throw it up/numb it maybe I can make it go away." Guide them in becoming a parent and caregiver to that part of themselves that is experiencing shame and help them offer compassion to that part of themselves.

Reimagining Their "Reproductive Story"

This can be done with an individual or with a couple. Process the "reproductive story" that they had in their minds, which starts from when they were little or the story they imagined about them ultimately becoming a parent one day: what they imagined when they were young, influences, and so forth, to where their stories got halted. Do some breath work and soothing guided visualization to ground them in their bodies. Once they feel grounded from the emotional trauma, they can start "trying on" new stories, which allows them to fantasize about what possible changes or new choices in the story could look and feel like. This involves a lot of acceptance work and self-compassion. These stories might be different from the original stories but can also be okay and true.

Probes in Mindfulness

Probes, contact statements, and little experiments are part of some common interventions in Hakomi therapy.[9]

Psychotherapy can be significantly deepened and expedited by using present-time experience in the assessment process and by incorporating experiential interventions.

What is a probe?

- A probe is an experiment done based in the present moment and in mindfulness.
- There are verbal and non-verbal probes; focus on verbal probes.

Probes are a way to go fishing for material to work with in session and often explore the memories and beliefs that organize the client's experience.

Probes come from what we learn progressively about our client. We learn their "story" that they have told themselves or that they have been told about themselves.

We listen to the negative beliefs (core beliefs) that come up in a session. We sift through the words but also the gestures, tone of voice, posture, and so forth.

The probe may come from a *missing experience* (being picked up as a baby, physical touch by their caregiver, positive affirmations about who they are). We ask: what kind of nourishment did this person miss growing up?

What is the purpose of a probe?
—Bring to consciousness how a person is organized around a particular issue in order to study and explore it.

Ex: Boundaries: it's ok to say no.

—Clarifying barriers to nourishment.
Ex: I like your vulnerability.

—Introducing the possibility of new options (new perspectives).
Once you have explored the story behind their negative belief, repeat the probe (which can offer a new experience or possibility to them about themselves) and explore the part of the client that wants to, longs to take it in.

—Helping to integrate the work.
Later in therapy, can be repeated and explore around it, body, movement, memories.

How do you prepare to use a probe?
—Take time to prepare the ground for mindfulness. Go slowly.
—We ask the client to notice what happens, to note his/her reactions.

—Always explain the experiment before doing it.
—Lower tone of voice, slow delivery to let it sink, slow, soft voice.
—Offer a menu of possible outcomes (you may feel nothing at all, you may feel discomfort, you may feel warmth in your body, etc.). There is no right or wrong way to feel.
—Guide the client to pay attention to his/her inner life.
—Say it as a statement—matter-of-factly, with no convincing.

Process of using a probe with a client:
1. Ask client to become mindful, and guide them if necessary.
2. Wait till the client is ready. The client can signal you.
3. Offer a brief, simple statement (important, otherwise it becomes intellectual).

"Please notice what happens when I say to you . . ."
"What do you notice when you hear someone say . . ."

For people new to it, we expand:
"Please notice what you experience . . . it could be a thought . . . a feeling . . . a sensation or and image . . . a memory might come up or some tension in your body. It's doesn't matter which happens. If nothing happens, that's perfectly okay. You can signal me when you're ready."
Please notice what happens when I say to you. . .

PAUSE!
(Allows a moment to anticipate and prepare so that the client can notice more subtleties of the experience.)

After delivering the probe, we track for the client's reaction to it.
Goal: provide the missing experience, a nourishing statement.

Examples of probes:

You're a good person.
You're perfectly welcome here.
Whatever you feel is okay.
You are safe here.
I am here for you.
You can ask for what you want.
I'll listen to you.
You're important.
You can show me who you are.
Your life belongs to you.
You don't have to prove anything.
You're lovable the way you are.
It's okay to rest/slow down.
You can be your full self.

Some of these are very generic. They come up over and over for clients.

Others are very specific to the client's experience. Your creativity is the limit.

Probes have to be honest, realistic and truthful—not "you will never be hurt again."

Probes are nourishing or potentially nourishing, never harmful, and try not to use negative words such as "no, don't, not," and so forth.

We offer nourishment. We give the client the opportunity to take in something that's needed or to see clearly that he or she rejects what's offered.

From there we can explore how and why that nourishment is rejected.

That's where the growth potential is.

For a woman in recovery who is trying to get pregnant and experiencing fertility issues, a useful probe in mindfulness for her might be something like "You are whole" or "It's okay to feel pain and loss."

For a woman who is active in an eating disorder and feeling confusion, shame, guilt or fear, a useful probe for her might be "You don't have to do it yourself/alone." "You can do what you want and still be loved."

Therapists: Can you come up with more examples?

Miscarriage and Pregnancy Loss: Another Form of Infertility

Miscarriage and pregnancy loss are the "silent" losses, as they are called, but there is nothing silent about them. Pregnancy loss may evoke a visceral moan coming from the deep depths of the mother's soul. They can occur for many reasons, and frequently doctors do not know why. A woman most commonly may miscarry due to chromosomal defects in the embryo that would make the pregnancy unsustainable in the long term. Other medical complications and factors can also influence the sustainability of a pregnancy. Factors such as a medical condition for mom or baby, trauma to the mother's body during pregnancy, co-occurring substance abuse, or an active eating disorder can increase the chances of a miscarriage or pregnancy loss.

The term "miscarriage" unjustly and pejoratively implies that the woman mis-carried the child, suggesting that she is at fault and further internalizing the stigma and shame that can come with experiencing a miscarriage. This is one of the reasons that miscarriages, like eating disorders, are not talked about. It would be incredibly reparative for all women (and their partners) in this population if we could come up with a less blaming and narrow-minded word to describe this type of loss.

When public figures and celebrities open up about these types of uncomfortable topics like infertility (surprise! They are humans too and undergo struggles just like the rest of us), it truly helps to normalize the discussion and reduce shame.

In her groundbreaking new memoir *Becoming*, former First Lady Michelle Obama opens up about the miscarriage that she suffered over 20 years ago, and about how she and former President Barack Obama conceived their daughters Malia, now 20, and Sasha, now 17 through IVF. "I felt lost and alone and I felt that I failed," says Mrs. Obama. She now reflects on that time in her life and wishes that she had known other women who had experienced miscarriages, which might have helped to reduce the shame she felt. "I felt like I failed because I didn't know how common miscarriages were because we don't talk about them," Mrs. Obama explains.

> We sit in our own pain, thinking that somehow we're broken. That's one of the reasons why I think it's important to talk to young mothers about the fact that miscarriages happen and the biological clock is real because egg production is limited—I realized that as I was 34 and 35, and we had to do IVF. I think it's the worst thing we do to each other as women: not share the truth about our bodies and how they work and how they don't work.[10]

Mrs. Obama is hoping that by sharing her story, she can help alleviate some of the shame and guilt that women feel when they suffer a miscarriage.

While it is so healing for women who have experienced pregnancy loss to hear from others about their own journeys with miscarriage, why do women wait periods of time, sometimes years (or decades) to open up about it? Beth, 33, who has struggled with infertility, shares:

> I think it is happening more and more often [women opening up about their fertility struggles]. I also think that people open up over time, and not in the moment because it is just so intense and so raw—it's not that you want to be private, it's just that you can't keep coming undone every little second. Wanting a child and not being able to conceive is a vulnerable and powerless feeling unlike any other—it's just such a primal impulse. And losing a child that you feel so hopeful about, at a time when those around you don't even know that he or she was with you is so very isolating. So much love to all the women struggling.

For a woman who is fully recovered from an eating disorder, like myself, to undergo two subsequent miscarriages with unknown causes can trigger a feeling of out-of-control loss. Many of the women I interviewed also experienced miscarriage, and some of them multiple losses. A common factor that several of these women described was being active in their ED while pregnant and the lack of sustained nutrition, the dehydration, and the weight fluctuations (some of them significant) affecting their growing fetus. A growing fetus needs more fat, carbohydrates, and complex nutrition than a woman's body would need to be healthy prior to becoming pregnant. Eating disorder behaviors during pregnancy, such as chronic restriction, bingeing and purging, laxative abuse, or excessive exercise, can put her baby at risk of not getting the sustained nutrition it requires to develop into a healthy child.

Going back to the research, we know that our "caveman brain" wants to protect the body by any means possible if it perceives a risk of starvation or death. An eating disorder can threaten the health of the body, and if it feels there are not enough resources to grow a baby *and* keep the woman alive, it may terminate the pregnancy so that the body can survive. This is a devastating trade-off but one stemming from our ancestors to preserve the future of the human species. The stress of an eating disorder on the body can also override the equilibrium of the system and put the woman at risk for her body rejecting the pregnancy.

A surprising result discovered in my research is the high rate of miscarriage and pregnancy loss in women with binge eating disorder (BED). Linna et al. have performed one of the few studies on this topic. They found that for most patients with BED, they are somewhere on the spectrum of obesity, which is known to have an adverse effect on reproductive health, including miscarriage. In their 2013 study of women who have eating disorders and are pregnant, they found that 50% of their participants who had BED suffered a miscarriage. This is higher than the rate of non-ED women who have miscarriages and the rate of women who have bulimia or anorexia, although these disorders contribute to higher rates of miscarriage than average as well. Lashen et al. have suggested that perhaps the effects of PCOS, diabetes, endometriosis, oocyte abnormality, or high insulin, which are all associated with obesity, may cause detrimental effects on a woman's pregnancy. Other complications such as elevated stress hormones related to binge eating, leptin, and adiponectin (protein hormones that help regulate glucose levels and break down fatty acids) abnormalities, dietary factors, hypertension, and cardiovascular disease may also contribute to fertility issues.[11] With the amount of weight stigma in our society, the impact of implying being in a larger body may trigger a miscarriage can add to the already present shame of someone who has miscarried. More research and understanding is warranted.

Polycystic Ovary Syndrome

Polycystic ovary syndrome, or PCOS, is an endocrine disorder affecting 6%–18% of reproductive-age women, with up to 69% of women being undiagnosed. Symptoms might include menstrual irregularities, high levels of testosterone, acne, excessive hair growth, obesity, and ovarian cysts. PCOS is a genetic disorder and symptoms may emerge right around the time a woman gets her first period or not until later in life after she has gained weight as a symptom. Many women do not receive a diagnosis of PCOS until they try to get pregnant.[12]

Research on the link between eating disorders and PCOS is complicated, in process, and sometimes contradictory. A significant study has shown no significant link between PCOS and eating disorders, although emotional distress resulting from a PCOS diagnosis could trigger ED symptoms, especially if weight loss is the primary medical recommendation. The diagnosis of PCOS was also found to contribute to self-esteem issues and self-isolation.[13]

A separate study found that PCOS has been associated with bulimia nervosa. It found that 75% of patients studied with BN also had PCOS and about 33% with PCOS having bulimic symptoms. It also found a link between BED and PCOS, although more research is needed on this connection. Interestingly, it found that higher rates of androgens in a patient, which is a symptom of PCOS, leads to higher rates of testosterone in this population, which stimulates appetite and is linked to poor impulse control, irritability, and depression.[14]

Insulin resistance, which is the primary factor of PCOS, occurs with and without obesity in women with PCOS, and lifestyle modification interventions aimed at improving insulin sensitivity rather than a weight focus are most effective, especially if the patient is prone to shame or disordered eating patterns.

A full screening of eating disorders needs to be done by a medical provider before suggesting weight loss for PCOS. More research is called for with this diagnosis, especially around the link between PCOS and shame. For some of the women I interviewed, they shared feeling judgmental toward their bodies once again for "not functioning correctly" and experienced guilt as if they had contributed to the disorder, even if research supported it being genetic. PCOS is the leading cause of infertility in industrialized nations and can threaten to stand in the way of a woman and her dream to have a baby, and yet many women with PCOS are getting pregnant through fertility treatments or without intervention.

Secondary Infertility

Secondary infertility is defined as "the inability to become pregnant or to carry to term a baby or after previously giving birth to a baby." Secondary infertility affects 12% of women and shares some of the same factors as primary infertility (the inability to get pregnant and carry a baby to term the first time).

Among the possible causes of secondary infertility are:

- Impaired sperm production, function or delivery in men
- Fallopian tube damage, ovulation disorders, endometriosis, and uterine conditions in women
- Complications related to prior pregnancy or surgery
- Risk factor changes for you or your partner, such as age, weight, and use of certain medications.[15]

For a mother who has a history of an eating disorder, what is the correlation between experiencing primary and secondary infertility? I did not find much data on this topic, but through my own qualitative research I have learned that instances of postpartum depression or anxiety can increase the stress about having a second child. Many women have symptoms of post-traumatic stress disorder (PTSD) after experiencing infertility and go through tremendous fear, guilt ("survivor's guilt"), worry, and uncertainty about trying to conceive another child.

"What if it happens again?" "What if I can't conceive?" "What if I conceive and experience another pregnancy loss?" "I don't think I can bear that": these are the voices of women in this population. This also sets them up to experience further shame if they find they struggle to get pregnant or do experience a pregnancy loss. Is this due to my ED history? Is there something wrong with my body?

Lacy, 36, is a married mother of a 5-year-old daughter. Lacy has been in recovery from anorexia since 2002 and experienced primary infertility when trying to conceive her daughter. Going through fertility treatments that were not successful, she and her husband William eventually got pregnant naturally with their daughter: it was a miracle, she says.

> The second time we decided to try to get pregnant I told my husband that I didn't want to do any fertility treatments and if we couldn't

get pregnant "naturally," I was happy with our family of three. We began trying before our daughter turned 2 years old and for over a year, we didn't get pregnant and I had mixed emotions. In the beginning, I was excited and hopeful about getting pregnant. My reproductive endocrinologist had said she thought we wouldn't have any problems the second time once my body "knew what to do." As time went on and we didn't get pregnant, I began to experience feelings of shame, anxiety, and depression again. I questioned myself a lot and also struggled with feelings of guilt and self-doubt. My husband really wanted a second child and I didn't feel the urgency I had before and wasn't sure what measures I was willing to take to get pregnant. I wanted to live our life and be present with my daughter. I didn't want to be consumed by trying to get pregnant again. We had a lot of discussions about what we were and were not willing to do.

A little after a year into trying, I found a new OBGYN and when I met with her she suggested I start tracking my cycle again and said she'd prescribe progesterone since it seemed to help the first time. When she said I'd have to track my cycle in order to take the progesterone, I felt panicked. I didn't want to start tracking again because I was afraid it would be all consuming and I didn't want to deal with the emotions I experienced the first time. I left the appointment still unsure of what I was and wasn't willing to do. The day after the appointment, I had a panic attack thinking about it. I decided to return to therapy to try to clarify my feelings and how I wanted to move forward. My husband and I had many conversations and unlike the first time, were in two different places. He wanted me to track my cycle and try the progesterone and I didn't. Yet I worried about regrets and experienced guilt at the same time. I decided to get the Ava bracelet (a fertility tracking bracelet) since it was very easy to use and would require little effort on my part to track my cycle. I started tracking my cycle in December and decided to wait on trying progesterone again to see how things would go. I experienced more anxiety wearing the bracelet and being so plugged in to what my cycle was doing and also found that each time I ovulated and didn't get pregnant, the disappointment and shame showed up again. It was difficult but I also knew that if I didn't really give it a true "try" by tracking my cycle, I might always experience feelings of guilt and regret. Once again, I turned to my values for guidance. I was also motivated by my husband's desire for a second and my daughter's desire for a sibling. I was constantly reflecting on how to balance my needs and boundaries with my family's needs and desires. After a few months of tracking my cycle, I decided I didn't want to take the progesterone and didn't know if I wanted to actively "try" anymore.

> After a very emotional and difficult counseling session, I told my husband I didn't think I wanted to try anymore and he was very sad but understanding. We felt a loss after this, although because we didn't know what that meant. Should I keep wearing the Ava bracelet? Did this mean we were going to avoid having sex during the time I was likely ovulating, etc.? Or should we continue not trying to prevent getting pregnant and see what happened? We had numerous difficult and emotional conversations and didn't come up with the answers to these questions. While we were having these conversations, I kept wearing the Ava bracelet at night mainly because I was unsure of what to do and it was habit. I knew I was going to ovulate soon and decided not to put any pressure on it (or at least try not to). My husband also knew I was going to ovulate soon. When I saw I had ovulated, I knew there was a possibility I might get pregnant but didn't expect it. A few weeks later I started having symptoms and knew I was pregnant. I tested at 4 weeks and it was positive. I was very excited and somewhat surprised by my excitement after all we had been through! I knew I had wanted a second child years ago and I think I had convinced myself it wasn't going to happen and not allowed myself to hope or want it anymore as a form of self-protection. I know I would've accepted only having one child if that had been our journey but it turns out it wasn't.

Lacy's experience highlights the fear, shame, and anxiety that secondary infertility can bring, as well as the brain's way of protecting her from those exact things: she had convinced herself that she wasn't going to get pregnant again and tried to not allow herself to feel hope. When she and her husband decided to stop actively trying, this is when she did conceive, perhaps due to the reduction of pressure on them. This occurrence is fairly common in couples who try to get pregnant for so long and it becomes something that is anxiety producing and stressful; they find that by taking the focus and intensity off of conception that they actually have an easier time getting pregnant.

A note: many people trying to get pregnant are told by well-meaning friends and family: "Just stop putting so much pressure on yourself!" "Relax and it will happen!" This can be invalidating to the couple, as it is not easy to just "stop stressing" about something that matters so much to them and carries so much weight. In this case it can be difficult to know how to respond to family members who may themselves be feeling stress about the situation. Setting boundaries and focusing on self-care are solid and effective options for perseverance in this type of situation.

The intersection of secondary infertility and eating disorders requires more research, and factors such as sperm health can affect fertility and not be related to a woman's ED.

Another case study brings to light the effect of BED on primary and secondary infertility. As discussed in the previous section, studies have shown higher rates of miscarriage and pregnancy loss in BED than in other eating disorders. Hilary, 40, struggles with depression and has a history of disordered eating since age 12, starting off as restriction and cycling to bingeing and some purging/laxative abuse. Since age 20 it has primarily shown up as bingeing and emotional eating.

> My husband and I tried to conceive for 1½ years before IUIs (3 times) and IVF (once) to get pregnant with my now-5-year-old daughter. We tried IVF to achieve pregnancy for Baby #2 without success. During this process I experienced two miscarriages; one loss at 5 weeks after a FET (frozen embryo transfer) and one loss at 7 weeks after IVF ("fresh cycle," not frozen). This was the hardest time of my life.
>
> I don't think that my past with an eating disorder affected my fertility, although I do sometimes wonder about this and feel guilt. I never became severely underweight and I never have been obese (have been overweight but my weight was never mentioned by fertility doctors to assist/affect my success). I was able to follow all the dietary guidelines by fertility doctors in order to make sure my pregnancy with my daughter was healthy and I ate enough, didn't over-exercise.

Hilary is still coping with the loss of being able to have a second child. She has entered intensive outpatient treatment for her eating disorder and is feeling solid in her recovery. While her doctors could never define the reasons for her infertility and called it "unexplained," there are still questions remaining about if her infertility is related to her eating disorder.

Women With an Active Eating Disorder Who Get Pregnant

Within this group there is also the category of women who have active eating disorders and who want to get pregnant, but are desperately struggling with their ED recovery at the same time.

Micali's recent study of women with eating disorders and their fertility challenges found that about 8% of pregnant women have an eating disorder. Only two studies to date have been done examining women with eating disorders attending fertility clinics, and those have found a high prevalence (16%–20%) of current EDs in that population. We also know that only about one-third of women will tell their OB/GYN if they have a current or past ED.[16] These data points show that eating disorders can have a significant impact on a woman's reproductive health, causing them to struggle to successfully conceive and carry to term a baby more than they might have if they had not had an eating disorder.

One of the significant effects of both AN, BN, and often BED is amenorrhea, which is the loss of a menstrual cycle. Women who have a severe active ED have reduced fertility and lose their menstrual cycles, and in some cases with AN, amenorrhea continues even after recovery. It is also found that amenorrhea or oligomenorrhea (irregular menstrual cycles) were present in 60% of women with BN, even if these women were at a normal weight.

A symptom of an eating disorder is the irrational thought that "I am above all normal rules; they do not apply to me." For me, anorexia gave me the idea that if I didn't eat, I didn't have to feel the intense emotions I was experiencing. Bulimia gave me the idea that if I binge and purge, I don't have to suffer the "consequences" of the binge (emotional and physical, such as weight gain or shame). My magical thinking kept me in a form of chaos, rigidity, and avoidance that quickly spiraled out of my own control despite my distorted belief that I was in control. The irrational thoughts led to irrational behavior such as stealing food and hiding it that took me further and further away from my own values and my sense of self.

Risky behavior such as binge drinking, drug use, stealing and lying, erratic driving, and other "rule-breaking" behaviors are common with AN, BN, and BED, and most frequent in BN. Since amenorrhea is a symptom of AN and also is common in BN and BED, women may believe they are not able to conceive and reduce or stop their use of contraceptives during sex. This can be seen as another risky behavior.

In Micali's study of unplanned pregnancies in women with an eating disorder versus those without any mental health illnesses, it was found that the prevalence of unplanned pregnancies was higher among all ED groups than in those without an ED or mental illness. The term "lifetime" is used when an eating disorder is chronic and spans the majority of a person's adult life without significant periods of recovery.

This study found that unplanned pregnancies occurred at a rate of 32.3% for women with lifetime AN, 25.3% for women with lifetime BN, and 32.3% for women with lifetime AN and BN as compared to women without mental disorders, which had an unplanned pregnancy rate of 22.3%. Furthermore, women who had AN the year prior to getting pregnant reported the highest rate of unintentional pregnancy (55.2%), giving the impression that they might have believed they could not get pregnant and did not use any form of birth control. As Jennifer Gaudiani, a prominent internal medicine doctor and eating disorder specialist in Denver, says, "eggs happen," even if a woman has skipped her period, a phenomenon called intermittent ovulation.

Of the women with AN or BN in Micali's study who became pregnant unintentionally, only 30%–40% reported being pleased with the pregnancy. They reported more than any of the other groups having mixed feelings well into the second trimester. Women with lifetime AN reported having five times the odds of increasing mixed feelings about being pregnant into the second trimester.

This subgroup of women goes through an intense identity "crisis" once finding out they are pregnant. Many women report a negative attitude toward pregnancy due to fear of losing their "anorexic" (or ED) identity, uncomfortable body changes, and adopting a new role of mother.[17] For a woman who struggles to take care of herself due to her ED, it is overwhelming and dangerous to put her in a position of needing to take care of another (helpless) being.

In addition, there is a group of women who are still struggling with their ED, whether they are fully involved with it or doing treatment and are in partial recovery, who strongly desire to have a family. I interviewed several of these women who fought so hard to do what they needed for their bodies in order to get and stay pregnant.

Olivia, age 33, is now the mother of two young children. She has struggled with body image and was on a diet that eventually developed into eating disorders at the age of 10. Her doctors informed her that she needed to gain weight in order to be healthy enough to carry a baby and also to hopefully get the return of regular menses, which she had not consistently had for over a decade.

Olivia reported trying her best to fight off ED thoughts and to follow the guidelines of her nutritionist to gain weight but also found herself engaging in the binge/purge cycle several times before she got pregnant. When she did get pregnant with the use of progesterone, she felt a mix of emotions. She stated:

> I really made a conscious effort to be careful with my body because I feared miscarriage and I constantly was aware of the fact that my body was no longer my body and that it was my responsibility to love/nurture/nourish my baby.

As she worked harder to fight off ED thoughts, the eating disorder identity that she had lived with for so long fought to retain its place in her life. She also engaged in ED behaviors periodically during her pregnancy, but not as often as she had earlier in her life.

Her first child was born 4 weeks premature and when she got pregnant again a couple of years later, she struggled even more intensely with coping with ED thoughts and behaviors than she had with the first. Olivia's second child was born 6 weeks premature and she endured a traumatic birth experience. This, on top of caring for a toddler and trying to keep up her house, job, and marriage, led to feeling overwhelmed. She tried to manage with counseling and other therapeutic support, but she also ended up relapsing in her ED.

While there are numerous sources for women to learn about childbirth and stages of pregnancy which paint these experiences in almost a magical way, what is not talked about nearly as much as needed are the multiple factors of stress and feeling overwhelmed that greet new parents the second their child is born and reality hits: how to feed the child, keep them safe, warm, and alive, while also trying to take care of yourself, your life outside of baby, and perhaps a second child like Olivia had. The list of new and evolving tasks for a parent never ends and can feel utterly overwhelming. More of this will be discussed in the postpartum chapter, along with more discussion about why ED relapse is so high in postpartum women with a current or past ED. As internal and external support can feel outweighed by the stress of incorporating another being (a fully dependent one) into one's life, it is not a big shock that the ED can creep back in.

Olivia tearfully stated to me:

> Looking back over the past few months since feeling ready to address some of the birth trauma from my most recent pregnancy, I strongly believe that my eating disorder stole my pregnancies from me and hindered my freedom to enjoy the amazing thing our bodies to do to create another human being and give life.

This speaks volumes to the toll that an ED can take on a person's well-being and their ability to adjust to life changes, and how shame can be such a significant underlying factor to the presence of an ED.

The narrative of Chloe, 32, shed light on yet another population of women, those with active eating disorders who experience pregnancy loss, whether intentionally through abortion or unintentionally through miscarriage. Chloe is now fully in recovery with three healthy children. She says her eating disorder hit official onset at age 11, but has had disordered eating since her father died when she was 8. She has had several hospitalizations, inpatient and outpatient therapy at several treatment centers, and periods of recovery for 15+ years.

Ballet and an abusive mother were maintaining factors in Chloe's ED. At age 18, she became pregnant unexpectedly and was forced into an abortion. She always longed to be a mother, and when she got pregnant again at 19 with the man who would become (and still is) her husband, she would not get an abortion again and settled down to raise a family overseas with him. Her eating disorder was quiet during her pregnancies, except one pregnancy where she was active in her eating disorder (restriction, overexercising, purging) and had a miscarriage. "I carry a great deal of guilt around miscarrying because I was intensely active in my ED at the time," she says.

Due to her husband being deployed for the first year of all of her children's lives, combined with being alone in a foreign country and not having a healthy attachment history herself, she struggled with postpartum depression (PPD) and her eating disorder spiraled out of control again after each birth.

> I remember (my firstborn) was about 2 months and wouldn't stop screaming. I felt full of rage; I laid him on the floor in the middle of the living room, shut the door and went upstairs to scream/ugly cry because I wanted to hurt him. In that moment I truly understood how moms get to the point of hurting their children.
>
> Therapy and showing up authentically in relationships has been the most healing experience for me. I didn't tell anyone about the screaming baby incident until many years later because I had so much shame around it. It wasn't until grad school that I understood the value in sharing my story.

Chloe's courageousness and resiliency through very tough situations and mental health problems have highlighted the efficacy of getting good support during the transition to parenthood and beyond.

Physical Triggers of Pregnancy

Physical symptoms of pregnancy may potentially have an adverse effect on a woman's recovery from her ED. Morning sickness, characterized by nausea and sometimes purging during the first trimester, may bring back memories of eating disorder days and behaviors. Throwing up from morning sickness can mimic throwing up from an eating disorder behavior, and this can cause complex feelings for a woman. Numerous women that I interviewed told me that even if they had been recovered for years, feeling an urge to throw up due to morning sickness was triggering old ED pathways in their brain. An eating disorder voice may say: "you can lose weight this way, or prevent yourself from gaining 'too much' weight during your pregnancy," or "doesn't this feel nice?" whereas there is nothing pleasurable about throwing up out of morning sickness. Also, purging in an eating disorder is done consciously and intentionally, where morning sickness occurs independently of the mom's control and can happen in the most unfortunate circumstances, like while driving her car or in a meeting at work. If a pregnant woman experiences a recurrence of disordered thoughts, she is encouraged to bring this up with her doctor and therapist and try to diffuse the unhealthy thoughts.

Digestive issues are common in pregnancy, such as constipation, diarrhea, and heartburn. These also are experienced often during the course of an eating disorder, and a pregnant woman may be tempted to use disordered behaviors to address them, such as purging, restriction, and laxative use. The body can also remember using these behaviors during an eating disorder and this can almost automatically trigger an ED-related thought. This is normal and okay (not a sign of relapse!), and can be overcome by letting the thought pass by and instead choosing a way to address the issue from a recovery mindset. It is advised that a woman experiencing these medical issues of pregnancy talk to her doctor about the best and safest ways to address them. A woman and her treatment team can sort out these feelings in her body and identify them as normal (if uncomfortable) symptoms of pregnancy. She may also recognize that these symptoms are temporary and will pass as her pregnancy advances and/or she gives birth.

If a woman is active in her ED she is at risk of further or more intense digestive issues during pregnancy, however if she is in recovery she should have normal digestion and experience no issues outside of "normal" pregnancy issues. Doing blind weights (where the woman does not see her weight) is also something that a woman can advocate for if she feels she may be triggered by seeing the number on the scale at her doctor's office. In addition, a woman who has a history of an eating disorder may feel triggered by advice about nutrition during her pregnancy. While it is important for her fetus to get sustained and balanced nutrition, a mother should listen to her own body and try to not get too wrapped up with "shoulds" in her diet. More about intuitive eating during pregnancy will follow.

Clinical Tool: Belly Stories and Acceptance

Here's a tool that Olivia and I utilized in counseling often during the course of her pregnancy. It begins by using mindfulness to guide the client into a presence-oriented and aware place.

Together with the client, try to identify the underlying feeling (or feelings) that she might be experiencing. The can be done by going through a list of emotions and letting them sit with her until she connects with one that fits. Delving into more of the context of her story can also help identify feelings and emotions.

In Olivia's case, she reports struggling with the ED identity and letting it go (although she desperately wants to because her value of having a family is much more important to her), and the shame of letting it in sometimes as a coping mechanism or "old pattern."

She identifies shame, guilt, fear, and worry as primary feelings during her pregnancies as well as after. She also has feelings of joy and love when she feels her body growing her babies.

When working with a client in this type of population, it can be very powerful to have them do some body connection and acceptance work. Here's how it can be done.

Have the client sit on the couch and place her hands on her belly (no matter what size it is/where she is in her pregnancy). Notice the way that she places her hands on her belly and have her describe this feeling and position: Is it protective? Is it loving? Is it uncertain? Is it detached?

Next, ask her to describe the stories she has heard in her life about what pregnancy "should" be like and list them. For Olivia, this brought up past narratives about "how her body 'should' look during and after pregnancy." Then have her describe how the ED talks to her about her body and her pregnancy. This might be something like, "It tells me that I am too fat this early in my pregnancy and that I need to 'slow down' the weight gain," or "it is already giving me pressure about how to have the 'perfect' birth story and then to lose the weight I gained as fast as I can. I will be 'disgusting' if I don't."

Here, pause and help the client connect with their body and describe what she is feeling now. She may report feeling stressed, anxious, fearful, angry, or guilty. Help her breathe through this and remind her that this is the influence of the ED.

The next step is to have her describe how she actually feels in/about her body and pregnancy. Here is also where you can bring in the values work that you have been doing with her (identifying her strong value of family). She may describe something like "I am overjoyed to be able to have a family. I am nervous and have some residual anxiety, but I am so grateful to be pregnant and to be starting the family I have always wanted to have," or "my body will have its own pregnancy journey that is my own. I may feel tempted to compare myself to others but I know that I am healthy and strong."

Notice the discrepancies in these accounts and help her process and find acceptance for her own pregnancy journey—not anyone else's.

A "New" Eating Disorder

Fogerty et al. performed a study on the effects of an eating disorder during the perinatal period (pregnancy to 2 years postpartum). In their qualitative research of women with an eating disorder who are pregnant, the biggest theme that came out was the task of "navigating a 'new' eating disorder." Then, postnatally, the women's biggest task was navigating a return to the "old" eating disorder and integrating that into her new experience with her body, her attachment with her child, and coping with numerous life and role shifts.[18]

Fogerty's study echoed results I found during my own anecdotal research on how a woman's ED changes during pregnancy. It makes sense clinically that the ED would shift and transform as the woman's physical body changes and her sense of "control" changes as well.

One of the biggest maintaining factors of an ED is body image, or a woman's subjective experience of her body—how she feels in it, how she perceives it, how she thinks about it, translating into how she treats it. If an expectant mother has an active ED, she may be at risk of her eating disorder creating more rigid and fearful thoughts about the inevitable body changes she will encounter the more threatened the ED feels. An example of this is seen in Trinity, a 26-year-old pregnant woman who has had a history of restriction and body image issues since she was 14. She is intensely fearful of gaining weight during her pregnancy and her ED voice gets louder and louder the further along she gets in her pregnancy and as her body changes. Her ED identity feels threatened by the arrival of a new identity: mother. In truth, the identity of mother is stronger and more resilient than an eating disorder identity, however the fight to let the mother identity take precedence may be intense.

In his study, Fogerty interviewed women whose ED "adapted" and became new and different as it experienced tumultuous change, "including feeling grotesque, a struggle over their changing body weight and shape, new feelings of losing control, and a tug-of-war over their desires to both stop and continue their eating disorder behaviours."[19] It's as if the ED morphs into a new version of itself that may touch on the woman's most present fears so that it can maintain its "relevance" in her mind.

For the majority of pregnant women with an ED or body image issues, they intentionally wanted to work on recovery and found they experienced a reprieve from their ED symptoms and in turn felt like they discovered a "body they could love." Women with an ED during pregnancy experience an intense roller coaster of emotions and challenges, often swinging between fear of losing their ED and trying to maintain it, and fear of harming their child and wanting to protect it. Understandably, these emotional battles and "tug-of-war" to follow value-based behavior can foster feelings of shame, self-judgment, and self-criticism and decrease feelings of self-worth.

In Fogerty's interviews, as their bodies grew and changed, women who have an active ED's body dissatisfaction grew. This group of women was more likely to perceive their body changes as "getting fat" or "feeling fat" instead of "this is an effect of the pregnancy." Women felt this most intensely in the beginning stages of pregnancy (first 3 months).

> My boobs changed first and automatically I thought "oh God I'm getting fat." It was the first three months, you know, when your body starts changing but not enough to look pregnant. So you look like you're getting fatter rather than being pregnant. So that bit was difficult, emotionally.[20]

The process of shifting away from the negative ED mindset that fears loss of control and focuses this on body shape and size, and more to the experience of "being pregnant," was a refreshing perspective change.

Clinical Tool: Perspective Shift

This tool is simple. It is designed to help the client identify when the ED is influencing her thinking and to offer a different perspective.

During pregnancy, especially the first trimester when the body is gaining weight and preparing to grow the fetus, an ED can feel intense body dissatisfaction and promote feelings of being "grotesque." When a client uses phrases that are self-damaging and shaming, such as "my boobs got big and lumpy and my stomach felt fat and flabby," the clinician can help reframe. "This is your body's way of becoming pregnant; your belly stores fat to prepare for giving nutrients and providing a safe home for your baby." Help the client come back to her values and validate her struggle. This is an intensely stressful and painful time for someone with an ED.

Conceiving a child is a miracle. The body needs to be in an optimal state for the egg and sperm to meet and develop an embryo. When a physical condition such as an eating disorder is present, the body is thrown into fight or flight mode, trying to keep itself functioning to the best of its ability given the threat of this disorder. As we have explored in this chapter, conception is complex when there is an active or past eating disorder, and the multiple factors that may influence a woman's physical recovery can complicate her ability to carry a child.

Shame, fear, and anxiety are prominent in both women who get pregnant while dealing with an eating disorder as well as those who are recovered but want to begin their family. How do we, as health professionals, best support women in any and all of these phases of life? We will continue exploring this in our next chapter of the pregnancy phase, and look at additional clinical tools that therapists can apply to ease the pain and allow emotional release from these struggles.

Conceiving a child while in an eating disorder or if a woman is fully recovered is a complex emotional and physical process. As this chapter has outlined, there are numerous factors that may impact the health of the fetus or mother as she conceives and is in early pregnancy. An eating disorder will never "go away on its own," and a mother may struggle with intense shame and guilt as she decides how to bring a new life to the world while also dealing with the effects of an ED. Therapists will encounter incredible self-criticism from this population, but will also notice the resiliency and strength that a woman encompasses as she can fight her ED to create the healthiest environment for her child: her womb. The 9 (actually 10) months of pregnancy present new challenges and learning opportunities for women, their partners, and their support team, which will be the focus of the next chapter.

Considerations for Therapists

1. What factors would you consider if assessing a client who has an eating disorder and presents for therapy saying that she wants to try to get pregnant?
2. What biases, assumptions, or countertransference may show up for you in working with a woman who is pregnant who has an ED?
3. What are the top three clinical needs to be addressed in working with a woman who has been dealing with infertility?

Notes

1. Costin, C. (2017). *8 keys to recovery from an eating disorder*. New York, NY: W. W. Norton.
2. Behavioral Change Models. (n.d.). Retrieved from http://sphweb.bumc.bu.edu/otlt/MPH-Modules/SB/BehavioralChangeTheories/BehavioralChangeTheories6.html
3. Statistics & Research on Eating Disorders. (2018, September 14). Retrieved from www.nationaleatingdisorders.org/statistics-research-eating-disorders
4. Kimmel, M., Ferguson, E., Zerwas, S., Bulik, C., & Meltzer-Brody, S. (2015). Obstetric and gynecologic problems associated with eating disorders. *International Journal of Eating Disorders*, *49*(3), 260–275. https://doi.org/10.1002/eat.22483
5. Home. (n.d.). Retrieved December 28, 2018, from https://connect.asrm.org/home?ssopc=1
6. Domar, A. D., & Kelly, A. L. (2004). *Conquering infertility: Dr. Alice Domar's guide to enhancing fertility and coping with infertility*. London: Penguin Books.
7. Robyn Mourning, MS, MFTC, Revolution Recovery Trauma Services.
8. Kate King, LPC, www.kateking.org
9. Weiss, H. (2015). *Hakomi mindfulness-centered somatic psychotherapy: A comprehensive guide to theory and practice*. New York: W. W. Norton & Company.
10. Obama, M. (2018). *Becoming*. New York: Crown Publishing Group.
11. Linna, M. S., Raevuori, A., Haukka, J., Suvisaari, J. M., Suokas, J. T., & Gissler, M. (2013). Reproductive health outcomes in eating disorders. *International Journal of Eating Disorders*, *46*(8), 826–833. https://doi.org/10.1002/eat.22179
12. Michelmore, K., Balen, A., & Dunger, D. (2001). Polycystic ovaries and eating disorders: Are they related? *Human Reproduction*, *16*(4), 765–769. https://doi.org/10.1093/humrep/16.4.765
13. Michelmore, K., Balen, A., & Dunger, D. (2001). Polycystic ovaries and eating disorders: Are they related? *Human Reproduction*, *16*(4), 765–769. https://doi.org/10.1093/humrep/16.4.765
14. Kimmel, M., Ferguson, E., Zerwas, S., Bulik, C., & Meltzer-Brody, S. (2015). Obstetric and gynecologic problems associated with eating disorders. *International Journal of Eating Disorders*, *49*(3), 260–275. https://doi.org/10.1002/eat.22483
15. Secondary infertility: Why does it happen? (2017, February 08). Retrieved December 30, 2018, from www.mayoclinic.org/diseases-conditions/infertility/expert-answers/secondary-infertility/faq-20058272
16. Micali, N., Simonoff, E., & Treasure, J. (2011). Pregnancy and post-partum depression and anxiety in a longitudinal general population cohort: The effect of eating disorders and past depression. *Journal of Affective Disorders*, *131*(1–3), 150–157. https://doi.org/10.1016/j.jad.2010.09.034
17. Micali, N., Simonoff, E., & Treasure, J. (2011). Pregnancy and post-partum depression and anxiety in a longitudinal general population cohort: The effect of eating disorders and past depression. *Journal of Affective Disorders*, *131*(1–3), 150–157. https://doi.org/10.1016/j.jad.2010.09.034
18. Fogarty, S., Elmir, R., Hay, P., & Schmied, V. (2018). The experience of women with an eating disorder in the perinatal period: A meta-ethnographic study. *BMC Pregnancy and Childbirth*, *18*(1). https://doi.org/10.1186/s12884-018-1762-9

19. Fogarty, S., Elmir, R., Hay, P., & Schmied, V. (2018). The experience of women with an eating disorder in the perinatal period: A meta-ethnographic study. *BMC Pregnancy and Childbirth*, *18*(1). https://doi.org/10.1186/s12884-018-1762-9
20. Fogarty, S., Elmir, R., Hay, P., & Schmied, V. (2018). The experience of women with an eating disorder in the perinatal period: A meta-ethnographic study. *BMC Pregnancy and Childbirth*, *18*(1). https://doi.org/10.1186/s12884-018-1762-9

3 Pregnancy

When you've been at battle with your body—whether currently or in the past—and you learn that you are pregnant, a magnificent wave of emotions surges through you. As quoted by author Elizabeth Stone, "making the decision to have a baby is momentous. It is to decide forever to have your heart go walking around outside your body."[1]

This elicits excitement, fear, joy, anxiety, anger, feelings of being overwhelmed, and so many more emotions.

I had the opportunity to talk with numerous women who finally got pregnant after many years of dealing with an eating disorder, and here is some of what they said: "I didn't know if this was ever possible for me; I am so happy!" "I am in disbelief. Do you think that I can actually have a healthy pregnancy? I have beat up my body so badly over the past ten years." "Is this real? What could go wrong?" The last statement came from a woman who had gone through 5 years of fertility treatments including three failed IUIs and two failed attempts at IVF. She had given up hope and had spent thousands of dollars to try to have a baby. She had struggled with anorexia for about eight years, has been in recovery for 3 years, and had utilized many forms of medication and nutrition support to try to get her body back to a healthy weight. It makes total sense that she has increased anxiety symptoms during the first few months of her pregnancy.

You may be thinking that getting pregnant is the best gift you could possibly experience after many years of struggling with yourself, your body, and food. And you are right—the gift of getting pregnant is unlike any other.

However, even for women who desire to have a family *so badly*, the changes that occur emotionally and physically during pregnancy may take them off-guard. Your body changes more rapidly when you are pregnant than at any other time of your life. In the first trimester, your body may once again feel as if it's against you, or you against it. Symptoms of early pregnancy include nausea, constipation, weight gain/bloat, dizziness, lack of appetite or increased appetite, and sleep disturbances, among other things. All of these are messages from your body to you, saying that it's working extra hard and trying to grow another human inside of it.

These changes continue during the length of the pregnancy as the child grows larger and stronger and begins to demand more and more energy, food, resources, and brain power from the mother's body. Pregnancy is also a time where women will get weighed by their doctor consistently and their weight will be monitored and discussed more than any other time of their lives. If the scale has been given absolute power over a woman's self-esteem, as may happen in the presence of an eating disorder, this focus on weight and numbers can be triggering and obsessive, especially if the woman's medical team overemphasizes the role of weight in fertility health (or any form of health).

Finding trust in your body and working to believe that it is telling you exactly what it needs to create a healthy baby may seem like an utterly foreign concept for someone who is struggling with an eating disorder. When a woman has dealt with infertility, as many of the women who I interviewed had done for years, getting pregnant and attempting to develop or revitalize that trust in their body can also be very challenging and wrought with loss.

While no one chooses to have an eating disorder, one can choose recovery for the first time or re-enter recovery if they have slipped. A woman and her partner can choose to start a family and yet once a woman is pregnant, there is so much out of her control that can be big triggers for her. A few of these are:

- Weight gain
- Food cravings or aversions
- Emotional mood swings and hormone fluctuations
- Nausea and morning sickness
- Stretch marks and growth of hips/breasts
- Back problems
- Forgetfulness, memory loss
- Exhaustion
- Insomnia/sleep issues.

Let's look further into the experience of pregnancy for both of our focus populations.

Women in Recovery Who Have Experienced Fertility Issues

I interviewed Michelle, a 27-year-old married woman who is mother to a 2-year-old boy and is newly pregnant with her second child. She had a 10-year struggle with anorexia and exercise addiction and currently defines herself as recovered, but says "it's not an on/off switch and is a long process of changing attitudes and behaviors." She adds, "I will always have a fragile relationship with food and my body." Her first pregnancy was unintentional, although she was very happy when she and her husband found out. She experienced a setback when she was diagnosed in early pregnancy with hyperemesis gravidarum, culminating in severe nausea and vomiting. This resulted in a drastic (yet unintentional) weight loss, which triggered some past ED thoughts: "When I was anorexic, I would get jealous of people who had an illness that caused them to lose weight." Her doctors are now focused on weight and numbers once again, as they had been when she was in treatment for her ED, yet this time for a different reason, which can require a huge mind shift. Michelle shares:

> I'm now pregnant again, this time after months of trying, but thankfully naturally. I probably stressed myself out about this more than necessary, but for a while I wasn't ovulating and assumed this had something to do with my ED past. I'm in my first trimester and still talk about this hesitantly, as if I could jinx a miscarriage, but I'm experiencing the same hyperemesis and weight loss as the first time. My ED past comes into view when I am pushed to eat more and increase intake, and purposefully think about what I am or not eating, or what I can or cannot keep down. I did purge previously, which changes the way your body deals with nausea and vomiting. I always used to think of vomiting as cleansing, and now every day I'm reminded of that ugly part of my past.

Some of the behaviors and conditions experienced during pregnancy can trigger past ED thoughts and memories, as happened with Michelle. Morning sickness may cause a woman to have the urge to throw up or she may actually throw up during this time in her pregnancy. Digestive issues, bloating, and body changes are common symptoms of eating disorders and also are common in pregnancy. Being aware of this connection and also of the very distinct difference between the triggering factors of these conditions can help a woman distance herself from her experience and notice that there is a productive (if uncomfortable) reason her body is doing this during pregnancy, while the opposite is true during an ED.

Intuitive Eating During Pregnancy—The Body Takes the Wheel

Intuitive eating is one of the most well-known and effective approaches for treating eating disorders, as it helps to reconnect the mind and body and focus on attuning to the body's inherent needs. It's the opposite of dieting or having rules around food and eating. Intuitive eating is an evidenced-based, mind-body health approach comprising ten principles and created by two dietitians, Evelyn Tribole and Elyse Resch in 1995. It is a weight-neutral model with a validated assessment scale and over 90 studies to date.[2] It incorporates a process called "interoceptive awareness" and helps cultivate connection and remove barriers to body awareness. Essentially, intuitive eating is a "personal process of honoring health by listening and responding to the direct messages of the body in order to meet your physical and psychological needs."[3]

You are the expert of your own body. Period. The physical and mental destruction of an eating disorder can make a woman feel that she has no control or power over her body and she turns against it. Through trying to eat intuitively, with no counting, numbers, tracking, rules, and so forth, a woman can learn to trust her body again, and her body can trust her again to give it what it needs.

Pregnancy is a time where the body's physical needs will assert themselves vehemently; the baby's survival depends on this. Intuitive eating is in a sense when the body takes the wheel. Here is a description of the ten principles of intuitive eating that may be helpful in working with any woman who has a history of disordered eating, and especially those in the prenatal period.

Ten Principles of Intuitive Eating

1. Reject the Diet Mentality:

   Get rid of the items that you have that talk about diets, of losing weight quickly, of the newest "trend" to "eat clean." Identify and challenge the rules and ideas you have been fed about this and how badly you felt when you gained back weight and lost self-esteem after each diet you have tried. Cleanse your life of diets; they are the opposite of intuitive eating.

2. Honor Your Hunger:

   Honor your hunger by eating what your body needs, fueling it with energy, carbohydrates, fats, and sugars. If you do not eat when you are hungry, you may trigger your body to biologically feel it is in survival mode and then eat mindlessly next time you do eat. It will take time to rebuild trust with your body and become aware of your hunger signals, but try to be patient and aware.

3. Make Peace With Food:

   Give yourself unconditional permission to eat and eliminate rules about "good" and "bad" foods. Again, if you restrict yourself or tell yourself you "shouldn't" have something, you will deprive your body which can trigger biological urges to eat the thing you "shouldn't." This may feel like a binge and can lead to guilt and shame.

4. Challenge the Food Police:

   Challenge the idea that you are "good" if you eat "good" food and "bad" if you eat "bad" food. The food police are deep in your psyche and are loud; you need to be louder. The food police always talks in rigid, all-nothing statements that are judgmental and guilt-inducing.

5. Respect Your Fullness:

   Listen for the body signals that tell you that you are no longer hungry. Observe the signs that show that you're comfortably full. Pause in the middle of a meal or food and ask yourself how the food tastes, and what is your current fullness level.

6. Discover the Satisfaction Factor:

   The Japanese have the wisdom to promote pleasure as one of their goals of healthy living. In our fury to be thin and healthy, we often overlook one of the most basic gifts of existence: the pleasure and satisfaction that can be found in the eating experience. When you eat what you really want, in an environment that is inviting and conducive, the pleasure you derive will be a powerful force in helping you feel satisfied and content. By providing this experience for yourself, you will find that it takes much less food to decide you've had "enough."

7. Honor Your Feelings Without Using Food:

   Find ways to comfort, nurture, distract, and resolve your issues without using food. Anxiety, loneliness, boredom, and anger are emotions we all experience throughout life. Each has its own trigger, and each has its own appeasement. Food won't fix any of these feelings. It may comfort for the short term, distract from the pain, or even numb you into a food hangover. But food won't solve the problem. If anything, eating for an emotional hunger will only make you feel worse in the long run. You'll ultimately have to deal with the source of the emotion and the discomfort of overeating.

8. Respect Your Body:

   Accept your genetic blueprint. Just as a person with a shoe size of 8 would not expect to realistically squeeze into a size 6, it is equally as futile (and uncomfortable) to have the same expectation with body size. But mostly, respect your body, so you can feel better about who you are. It's hard to reject the diet mentality if you are unrealistic and overly critical about your body shape.

9. Exercise—Feel the Difference:

 Forget militant exercise. Just get active and feel the difference. Shift your focus to how it feels to move your body, rather than the calorie burning effect of exercise. If you focus on how you feel from working out, such as energized, it can make the difference between rolling out of bed for a brisk morning walk or hitting the snooze alarm. If when you wake up your only goal is to lose weight, it's usually not a motivating factor in that moment of time.

10. Honor Your Health—Gentle Nutrition:

 Make food choices that honor your health and taste buds while making you feel well. Remember that you don't have to eat a perfect diet to be healthy. You will not suddenly get a nutrient deficiency or gain weight from one snack, one meal, or one day of eating. It's what you eat consistently over time that matters; progress not perfection is what counts.[4]

Drawing from these principles, it becomes clear that pregnancy is a time where your body is in the driver's seat and intuitive eating should be a natural response. Your body will tell you *exactly* what it does and does not need or want. For a woman who has recovered from an ED and applies intuitive eating in her everyday life, this way of eating might not seem so abnormal, although her pregnancy desires might be slightly different from her normal tastes.

Kendra, 29, who has had an 11-year off/on battle with disordered eating, expressed,

> When I was early in my pregnancy, I could not stand the smell of anything with much flavor in it. The smell of meat being cooked, the smell of garlic, anything that had a distinct smell made me feel sick. I had to learn that this was my body's way of coping with the hormone surges I was undergoing and that I should not try to override them. Later on in my pregnancy, I craved strange foods that I didn't eat very often in my normal life—like bananas, chili, microwave popcorn, edamame—random! It was such a strangely nourishing experience to trust my body that it would tell me loud and clear about its desires (sometimes changing hour by hour). Also, as the baby grows, your stomach and other organs get squished and lose space. I would eat and then be hungry again in the next half hour because my stomach just couldn't hold that much food at one time. When I was in my ED, this hunger surge would freak me out so much that I would probably restrict or get really critical of myself. Or my ED would think it's a "good thing" to have hunger and to let it grow. In

> pregnancy, there really are no rules about what your body might do and everyone's experience is vastly different. It kind of gives you the challenge of surrendering complete control and listening to your body.

As discussed earlier in the book, there is a high rate of remission of ED symptoms during pregnancy, as the mother may have a new "purpose" for trying to fuel her body and take care of herself. This also can mean that a woman may be eating more intuitively and less rule or fear based during pregnancy. This can be a positive learning experience as the mother learns new ways of nourishing herself, but can also be risky if the mother feels like she "knows how to eat intuitively" and loosens up her commitment to her eating disorder recovery. With a high rate of relapse of up to 70% by 18 months postpartum, there can be "magical thinking" during pregnancy that does not take into account the stressful reality of becoming a mother and caring for a newborn.[5] Pregnant women who have an eating disorder and want to practice intuitive eating may have a good chance of learning this during pregnancy and also need to be cautious about overconfidence.

Women With an Active Eating Disorder Who Get Pregnant

Another population of women are those who are active in an eating disorder and who get pregnant, whether intentionally or unintentionally. This experience also can have a huge emotional impact—both positively and negatively. As eating disorders are devastating to one's self-confidence, getting pregnant might instill a sense of hope or belief that one is worthy of being a parent, that they can try to recover for their child, or that they have a purpose much bigger than their ED. It also can bring up intense feelings of fear, shame, guilt, and anger for women who grapple with the changing roles and demands of pregnancy and impending parenthood. Some of the words I heard from women with EDs who got pregnant are "I felt angry that I had to stop or change my ED behaviors, I then felt incredibly guilty for feeling this way. I also felt ashamed for this battle I had inside of myself—who would choose an ED over their child? That's insane!" "The most common emotion I had was fear: how would I afford my ED and care for a newborn?" "Could I be present enough to care for a child?"

Pregnancy and becoming a parent initiate a tremendous and often stressful change to a woman's physical body as well as to her relationships and lifestyle. If a woman desires to become a parent, the best thing she can do for herself and her future child(ren) is to focus on fully recovering from her eating disorder before trying to get pregnant. Women who are fully recovered have the same chances of getting pregnant as a woman who has never had an eating disorder and a higher chance of delivering a full-term healthy baby than a woman who is active in her ED during pregnancy.[6]

Of the women who get pregnant and still struggle with an ED or disordered eating, a significant percentage of them (up to 60%–70%) decrease or eliminate completely their ED behaviors during the length of their pregnancy. This time can be described by women in this group as "magical" and "inspiring," and that "taking care of my child (through good nutrition, no/fewer ED behaviors, exercise, self-care, etc.) is more important than my eating disorder." This phenomenon is not replicated during any other life experience a woman with an eating disorder can go through. While it is wonderful that this group of women goes into remission during pregnancy, a risk that arises is that some believe they are "doing so much better with their ED recovery" and may terminate treatment with their counselor or dietician as they believe they don't need help anymore. It is not advised that anyone with an ED stop treatment during or after pregnancy, as the false phenomenon of perinatal recovery is incredibly dangerous.

For upwards of 75% of these women, partial or full relapse of ED symptoms will occur by 18 months postpartum. This is due to a variety of different reasons: stressors of tending to a newborn, old coping behaviors (ED being primary) resurfacing during stressful and transitional times, relationship stressors with their partner, financial demands of having a child, adapting to a different body and body image issues, recovering from birth, needing increased food intake to produce milk if they are breastfeeding, and much more.

Another subgroup of women reports that they "let go" during pregnancy and have described this to me as "not caring about what they eat, giving up rules, feeling out of control, gaining tons of weight." Many of the women who feel this way were "clean eaters" before pregnancy, meaning they followed a "healthy" diet, which in reality was often along the lines of a subcategory of disordered eating called *orthorexia*.

Orthorexia

Orthorexia nervosa is not officially included in the most updated diagnostic manual (DSM-5) but is emerging as one of the most common and mainstream forms of disordered eating. The term *orthorexia* comes from Greek words *orthos* (meaning "straight and proper") and *orexia* (meaning "appetite"). It is classified as the drive for "biologically pure food," meaning food that is free of toxins, dyes, chemicals, and so forth. People who begin this form of eating may initially do so in order to fight off disease, lose weight, or improve his/her health. However, this method of eating may become obsessive and ritualized, just as other eating disorders, and can lead to social isolation and negative affect, and the regimen of following the diet can become the most important thing in their lives.[7]

When they discovered they were pregnant, some of the women who had orthorexic behaviors realized they "couldn't" or "didn't have to" follow those strict health guidelines anymore, and in addition wanted their child to be healthy and getting the nutrition it needed. This was described as "a sense of relief." Others felt symptoms of panic and anxiety as they walked a tightrope between choosing recovery and choosing their eating disorder.

Sarah, 26, shares her story on her popular blog *Kiwi and Carrot*:[8]

> For the past ten years, I've been slowly killing myself. Weapon of choice? Kale and running shoes. No, really. This is true. The ironic part? I thought I was the healthiest human in the world. I was toned, I had a six pack, I never skipped my 5-mile daily run, and I did crunches and push-ups every night before I went to bed. I ate heaping piles of "lean protein" and vegetables and devoured berries, bananas and apples daily.
>
> People told me I was skinny, and complimented me on my ripped arms and quick WOD times in CrossFit. I could beat the guys at pull-up contests and I could hold a plank for 6 minutes straight. I was known as the fitness girl, and I was unstoppable. Occasionally I would wonder if I was pushing myself too hard. That maybe when I had a sinus infection or a pulled muscle I should skip my morning workout routine, but I was addicted. I was addicted to the rush of pushing myself physically and mentally, and I liked how I looked. I was comfortable with the number on the scale and I secretly felt proud of myself when I turned down a piece of cake because that meant I was healthy.
>
> My mind was sick. And so was my body.
>
> I hadn't had a natural period since I was 14, but I'd been on birth control for years, so I figured everything was fine.
>
> I began to have horrible digestion issues and was diagnosed with IBS and SIBO (small intestine bacterial overgrowth). Of course I didn't correlate this with my low weight and malnourished body. Instead I restricted further, cutting out gluten, dairy, sugar, all processed foods, believing that these were the culprits behind my gut distress. Things only got worse.
>
> When I went off birth control and didn't have a period, I got my hormone levels tested. My blood work came back reflecting the levels of a post-menopausal woman. I was 22. I was advised to get a DEXA scan to test for weakened bones because of the lack of estrogen in my body. That's when I learned that I had osteopenia. If I didn't do something to improve my bone strength, I would have osteoporosis at the ripe old age of 30. I was devastated and scared. I heard that weight-bearing exercise helped strengthen bones, so I increased my exercise, jogging the track while carrying 20 pound plates. I truly believed I was helping myself to heal.

I was able to sustain my rigid lifestyle for those 9 or 10 years, but then, at 23 years old, my body hit a wall. I started to have chest pain, weird heart palpitations. I wasn't sleeping well, my hair was thinning, I was anxious, stressed out and very unhappy.

And I wanted a baby.

But turns out you can't make a baby when you're infertile. "Fitness" had robbed me of my fertility. Instead of a baby I had six-pack abs, osteopenia and hypothyroidism.

I was broken.

After some Web MD-ing (I've gotten too familiar with that website) I diagnosed myself with hypothalamic amenorrhea (HA) and started researching. HA occurs when your hypothalamus (a region of your brain) senses that your body doesn't have enough resources to keep living. This can come from overexercise, under-eating, mental stress, or a combination of the three. In order to help you survive, your hypothalamus shuts off your reproductive organs, slows down your thyroid and down-regulates your metabolism. That way your brain and heart have enough energy to keep you alive.

Our bodies are so smart.

In my research, I learned that in order to reverse HA, I needed to make my body trust me again. I needed to gain weight and stop exercising. I needed to let my body have what it had been craving for years . . . food and rest. And lots of it.

I'm a very determined person, so I told myself I could do this. I sat on my bum and ate ice cream for two months. I cut all exercise besides walking and yoga. I gained 20 lbs. It was hard.

But I started to feel good. I had energy. My heart palpitations started to disappear. I felt a freedom I hadn't felt in years because I was no longer a slave to my morning workout routine. I no longer planned my day around my workouts, instead I did yoga if I wanted to and if I didn't feel like it, I'd skip that day.

It was hard to watch my body change. Good-bye abs, hello cellulite. My clothes didn't fit anymore, and I felt huge. But occasionally I would get a glimpse of my now slightly curvier body and think "hmm, this is how a woman is supposed to look."

I almost gave up, multiple times. When it had been 6 months and still no period, I started to slip back into my old exercise routine, figuring it was too late for me to get my fertility back. I had ruined my body and now I had to pay the consequences for my decisions.

But just as I was giving up for good, I stumbled on a book called *No Period, Now What?* by Nicola Rinaldi, PhD. It was just the push of motivation that I needed. With the incredible support of the online HA community and the knowledge and motivation the book offered, I decided to go "all-in" for a few more months and see what happened.

I took a deep breath, and settled in for the long haul. No exercise. Minimum of 2,500 calories a day.

Rinse and repeat.

I've been facing this fight for 9 months now and my battle is not yet over. I still have to wake up every. single. day. with the determination to eat ALL THE THINGS and don't stop till I've won. I know my body is waiting for me to get to its "happy weight" . . . the weight where it finally trusts me again. Only then will it give me my fertility back.

That day might come tomorrow, or it may come with another 20 pounds of weight gain. Only God knows my plan, so for now, I just wake up and try to face each new day with faith and a big bowl of ice cream. It's so hard to be patient. It's hard to trust the process and be ok with the weight gain. But I know it will all work out how it's supposed to.

True "health" and beauty are so much more than having 6-pack abs and wearing size 2 jeans. Whoever decided that was beautiful anyways? Just because society has put a stamp of approval on restrictive diets and skinny girls taking gym bathroom mirror selfies doesn't mean that's something we should strive for. I did strive for that and guess where it landed me? In the doctor's office with weak bones, infertility and a disordered mindset of what's healthy and beautiful.

Now I am the heaviest I've ever been in my life. I kissed my six-pack abs goodbye months ago. I had to throw out my entire wardrobe and I canceled my gym membership. (For now at least.)

But I am happier than I've ever been in my life, because now I am free. I no longer base my worth on how many calories I did or didn't eat, how many miles I did or didn't run or how my skinny jeans do or don't fit. Now I value myself because I am a daughter of God and a wife to an incredible husband. I am meant to be a mom someday and that's what really matters. I value and respect my strong body that is so, so forgiving and resilient. And I'm sorta thankful for the extra fat on my body because it means I am healthy, happy, and full of life.

I'm not saying I'm done with "fitness." Oh, heavens no! I will always love being active. Once my body is healed, I will continue to hike, run, lift heavy weights and rock climb. But now I have a much more balanced idea of what "fitness" looks like. It doesn't control me like it used to. Now I see fitness as a luxury that I get to enjoy when my body is rested and properly fueled. Everything has changed for me. And for those girls out there who are struggling with a toxic mindset of what "fit" and "healthy" is, I pray things can change for you too."

And Sarah's update a few months later:

I got my period back two weeks later (after my first story). First natural one in about 10 years! 40 days later I got a second period, and then a third.

After another month and another 10 lbs. of weight gain, my body finally got to its "happy weight . . ." the weight where it trusted me again. I got my first natural period I'd had in 10 years! I was thrilled. I'd worked SO hard to get to that point, and was finally rewarded . . . not just by the return of my fertility, but by a positive pregnancy test nine months later! After getting that first cycle back, I decided to give my body some time to build some bone mass back up and continue to heal and rest. I slowly added exercise back into my routine, and continued to have natural cycles for eight months, while maintaining my recovery weight. We got pregnant the first month we tried. . . . I think God decided I'd waited long enough.

I'm now 21 weeks pregnant with a little baby boy.

Looking back, sometimes I feel angry at myself for putting my body and mind through what I did for all those years. But then I remember it was all done in innocence. I never meant to harm my body. I'd just compared myself to my "skinny" friends and saw photos of "fit" people on Instagram and told myself I wanted that. I truly believed I was living a healthy lifestyle.

Oh how wrong I was.

So, for anyone out there struggling with what I've gone through, you can take encouragement from my experience (along with hundreds of other HA recoverees. . .). Trust the recovery process. The doctors may advise against it. Time and time again, women have been sent home with a prescription for this med, or that supplement; merely band-aids that will cover up the problem.

You are not healed until you address the root cause. So what is the root cause?

Too much stress. Too many six-pack abs. Too much restriction, too much exercise. Not enough food, not enough rest, not enough love for yourself and your body.

So there you have it. All the answers. Until doctors become more educated on HA, you may have to take your health into your own hands.

Several women interviewed from the subgroup of women who struggle with orthorexia and do get pregnant described their pregnancy period as a "lapse" of their ED if they were not able to devote themselves to true recovery as Sarah had. These women felt stressed about how to get their "pre-baby body back" and return to the optimal state of "health" as defined by their ED in the postpartum period. The weight gain during pregnancy is almost always described as "uncomfortable" and "temporary," and after birth this group of women is apt to return quickly to their "diet plan."

I have had multiple clients who come to me years after having children because they still struggle with body image and some disordered eating habits. It is common for them to describe their pregnancy experience(s) in this way—feeling out of control during pregnancy, then quickly dedicating themselves to return to their pre-baby body postpartum. Without addressing the underlying factors that perpetuate the diet/binge mentality, these women will continue to cycle through feelings of shame, guilt, empowerment, fear, and relief.

Pregorexia is a dangerous mix of pregnancy and orthorexia, and although also not officially included in the DSM, it is a widespread problem that occurs frequently and is not often discussed. Open up a popular magazine or visit a website that features celebrities or popular trends. You are likely to find pictures of pregnant women or new mothers, many of them discussing their "post baby" diet plans or "how they stay fit" during pregnancy.

It's important to have a clear delineation here: women are scrutinized their entire lives for their bodies, for their life choices—like if she wants to be a parent or not. By the time she is in her mid-twenties, a woman will get questions about getting married and having babies, as women are biologically "programmed" to do. If a woman does choose to get pregnant and is successful, she may devote herself to a healthy lifestyle for herself and her child to prevent pregnancy-related health issues like diabetes, preeclampsia, and other conditions.

The choice to be healthy during pregnancy is vastly different than a woman who has a disordered relationship with food and whose eating disorder harms her body instead of helps it during this time. Women may feel pressure to "stay fit" or "be active" during pregnancy, which when intertwined with anxiety, can lead to a dangerous condition called pregorexia. Pregorexia will be further discussed in Chapter 5.

The effect of pregnancy on a woman who has had a disordered relationship with food is intense and can go multiple directions, including how it might impact her identity. For women whose identities are closely connected with their body image and may have a career that involves attention on bodies/weight/food, this can be complex especially if they really value their career.

One client, Gina, 37, is a fitness instructor at a popular gym in town. She has had two children and described her pregnancies as "somewhat stressful, somewhat relieving" to not have to focus so intensively on keeping up the "fitness image" that she has carried with her since she was a teenager as part of her identity. She states that she gained "a lot of weight" during pregnancy and felt pressure to take it off as quickly as she could after birth. Now, 3 years after her second child was born, she is relapsing into her past eating disorder (bulimia), which she struggled with from ages 15 to 22. Gina feels pressure to try to maintain her weight and shape, as her identity as a well-known fitness instructor is tied to that. She also values health and fitness and wants to be "healthy," but feels so much shame at her hidden ED behaviors which are the complete opposite of healthy. Gina disclosed that she felt she lost some of her identity when she became a mother, which is a frequently utilized description by new mothers. She is her children's primary caregiver while her husband works long days, and she loves being there to care for her young family. It is also during the times when she is alone in the house or with her kids solo that she feels the urge to binge and purge. In therapy, she explored many pieces of her identity that she felt were lost or pushed down in her role as mother. The ED helped her cope with this sense of loss, and Gina explored her ambivalence to give it up due to the way that it helps her feel less lonely and isolated. She felt grateful that her husband is able to financially provide for the family, but also some resentment and jealousy that he is able to focus so intently on a career that brings him a great deal of confidence and worth.

Gina's experience echoes that which many mothers feel when the family must decide how to provide for children and if this means one parent staying home to care for the children. Many women love this incredibly demanding job. Some call it "thankless" or "invisible" and struggle with the shift or loss of identity that they may face, making them more vulnerable to self-destructive coping mechanisms such as disordered eating or substance use.

An approach that has been effective in working with clients like Gina incorporates the power of metaphor and mindfulness.

Clinical Tool: Metaphor, Meaning, and Moving Through the Mind's Monsters

The mind is a powerful mechanism. An eating disorder lives in a woman's mind and unabashedly drives the mind to disconnect from the body. In pregnancy, a woman is called to be fully present in her body, ideally without the presence of ED behaviors, which means she needs to learn to tolerate uncomfortable feelings and work to protect her body from the ED mind's viciousness.

A tool that I use with women who are at any point in their pregnancy journey is one that calls upon metaphor to help them ground in their bodies and untangle from the mind. We get out a large piece of construction paper and markers or get out magazines full of pictures. I direct the woman to draw her body as she sees it now. Then she uses markers and/or magazine clippings to create a metaphor of what she feels in her body. One client drew a sea of violent waves and menacing sea creatures in her belly, symbolizing the chaos that she feels in her stomach right now. In her womb she drew a protected vessel, holding her baby inside, navigating the intense highs and lows of the sea's temperament. She colored bright red the parts of her body that have changed the most in the pregnancy—her hips, her breasts, her thighs. She drew red pockmarks all over her face where she has developed pregnancy-related acne. She told me these were the "shunned spots," the places that her mind liked to focus on and judge harshly because they changed so rapidly, filling out with fat. Red symbolized anger, hostility, disgust.

I asked her to sit with this drawing for a bit, to close her eyes and put her hands over it, to breathe, and then to ground herself in her body, bringing her attention to the places that she had colored and decorated on the picture. My client said,

> I feel warmly toward that vessel that is trying to ride out the waves in that turbulent sea which is my belly. I am having a really hard time understanding why my body had to get so much fatter in order to help that vessel grow. In my mind, those two things are not connected and should not be. I know rationally that I am gaining weight as a normal part of pregnancy, that my baby needs the fat on my body to grow.

After she gave birth, my client struggled to accept her "changed" body for a very long time. We did the collage exercise again, and this time she colored her vessel outside of her body, a boat with her baby in it safely. In her belly were broken pieces of a different boat, which she described as "my body trying to sort itself out again. My organs got pushed all over the place by the baby and they are trying to find each other again in the calm after the storm." She was able to have more compassion for her body at this point, noting that it had "weathered a giant hurricane" and needed time and rest to restore itself.

We did this exercise regularly as she recovered postpartum and observed how her experience in her body got more accepting and more grounded as she focused on it in a more open way.

An Unintentional Parent

If a woman's pregnancy was not intended or desired, receiving news of conception may be a disruptive and triggering experience for the mother and/or for her partner. Many women who struggle with AN describe it as a "struggle" and have "anger at giving up their anorexic identity." They can feel resentment toward their baby, the baby's father, and themselves during the pregnancy which can increase the chances of the mother experiencing PPD or postpartum anxiety (PPA). Anxiety affects approximately 6% of pregnant women and 10% of women in the postpartum period. It can be experienced alone or comorbidly with depression. Symptoms of PPA include: constant worry; feeling that something bad is going to happen; racing thoughts; irritability; disturbances with sleep and/or appetite; restlessness; physical symptoms like dizziness, nausea, and racing heart; among others.[9]

In this population, negative attitudes toward pregnancy were more common than for women who described an intentional journey to pregnancy. This ambivalence can be related to the impending weight gain, the perception of lack of control, and the unexpected discovery of being pregnant. A recent study also found that positive attitudes toward pregnancy by someone close to the pregnant woman or by a therapist can have a beneficial impact on a woman with an ED and alter her perception of motherhood and her pregnancy.[10]

Jill was 26, drinking heavily and acting out on ED behaviors (bingeing and purging, restriction, and excessive exercise) three to four times per week. Jill had struggled with an ED since she was 14 and had periods of remission which had always been followed by periods of relapse when she encountered a big life transition or challenge. Alcohol abuse and her ED went hand in hand. She was in a relationship with Shawn, which was rocky and unstable. She had inconsistent menstrual cycles since she was a teenager and consistently "forgot" to take her birth control. During our work together, she was really focused on her career and wanting to recover from her eating disorder. Her relationship with her body was so damaged by the years she had struggled with her ED that she disconnected from it and abused it in order to "not feel" the pain that it held. She came from a family system of addiction and avoidance and felt that she could not get herself out of the grasp of the family cycle.

Jill skipped her period for a couple of months, but reported to me that this "was not uncommon for her." She was drinking daily and having struggles in her relationship with Shawn, but she was able to perform well at work. She also had two DUIs from a few years prior that she was still involved with legally. Jill reported feeling bloated, which again was not unusual for her given her ED history.

Then she came into my office one day in a complete panic mode: "I'm pregnant, Kate. I'm five months pregnant!" she said with tears in her eyes. She felt angry at Shawn, angry at herself, angry at her body, and very, very afraid. She was afraid she had hurt her baby through her ED behaviors and by drinking without knowing she was pregnant. She didn't know what to do.

She and I processed this a lot and she went to the doctor to get checked out. The doctor said from as far as she could tell the baby was healthy (heartbeat, size/weight, growth, etc.). Jill immediately stopped drinking but still struggled periodically with bingeing and purging. She was nervous because she "had been restricting and running 6–8 miles a day up to that point in her pregnancy."

Jill's first plan was to get a late-term abortion, as she did not know if she was ready to be a mother or if she "could do it." Shawn was not a positive influence on her or her recovery, and she was not where she wanted to be in her career and with little money saved. She discovered that there were only two doctors in the state who would perform this type of procedure. It was very expensive and would be very devastating to her body, let alone her conscience.

Through tears and panic, Jill tried to decide what was the best thing to do. Shawn was completely shocked by the news of her pregnancy and shut down, shut her and everyone else out, which contributed to Jill's shame, anger, and pain. Shawn came from a strictly religious family which he feared would not approve of the situation. He withheld the news until it was inevitable for them to find out, lacing more shame into his and Jill's relationship. They got in heated arguments fueled by the stress of the situation and the panic they both felt. This put added stress on Jill's body and on the baby she was growing.

After going through much counseling, soul searching, and pro and con lists, Jill then decided she wanted to put her baby up for adoption as she proceeded with her pregnancy. She contacted an adoption agency and was matched with a married couple who had struggled with infertility for years and wanted to adopt a child. Jill met with this couple, really liked them, and felt positive about her choice to give her child (her baby girl) to them. She really envied the relationship they had, which she felt was close, respectful, and loving . . . all of which she felt like she was missing with Shawn.

> They were very loving and involved in the process—they came to doctor's appointments, checked in on me constantly, and absolutely deserved to become parents. I remember really envying their relationship. With the decision of adoption I started taking care of myself like I had not done in a long time. I ate well—breakfast, lunch, dinner, and lots of healthy snacks. My ED seemed to be silenced because I was taking care of this little baby and that was more important than how I looked. And I really enjoyed being pregnant. I stayed active the entire pregnancy and it felt really great to fuel my body.

Meanwhile, Jill's family was also in a state of shock and were giving her mixed messages. Her mother encouraged her to keep the baby. Her father (who was divorced from her mother) wanted to her do what was best for her. Jill was torn. We did a lot of self-compassion work around this, trying to find a way to radically accept what her situation was and do the best for herself and for her baby. This was very hard for Jill, who was still having major difficulties in her relationship with Shawn. Shawn came from a Mormon family and he felt shame for the situation that they were in from a religious standpoint as well.

> One doctor's appointment at about 30 weeks changed everything. The nurse performing the ultrasound let it slip that the baby was a girl. I remember sitting in my car, staring at the picture and feeling like there was no way I could give up this little girl. After talking with several mentors and meeting with another mother who had gone through adoption with the same agency I made the decision

> that I was going to keep the baby. I told [Shawn] that he could walk away and not have anything to do with her or he could be involved but that I was going to keep her no matter what.
>
> It's hard to even write this because I cannot imagine life without her now.

Jill struggled with this decision so intensely—one year ago she could not imagine becoming a parent, and here she was deciding what to do with her soon-to-be-born baby girl. She felt awful for changing her mind and letting down the adoptive parents, who had had another mother change her mind at the last minute as well on top of enduring their own fertility losses.

Jill delivered a healthy baby girl surrounded by her family and Shawn. She looked at her healthy baby girl, who looked just like her.

She still struggled with body image and some ED behaviors (although these decreased significantly during her pregnancy) and wanted her baby to have a positive and healthy upbringing. Could she parent this child while also trying to recover and get her life back on track? She experienced fear of how she would raise this child, especially if she and Shawn were not together, and was on a wave of postpartum hormones.

It is necessary for me to do some self-disclosure here. During my time working with Jill, I was going through my own fertility journey. I had struggled to get pregnant for almost a year and had just suffered my first miscarriage when Jill told me she was pregnant. I then suffered a second miscarriage during our work together as well. At times it was a struggle for me to put my own pain aside to support her in her pain and angst. I was receiving supervision as well as my own therapy during this time. I speak to this because I think many clinicians go through personal life matters while they are working with a client who is going through something similar or somewhat similar but on a different path. We can feel surges of guilt for having our own emotions surface during the therapeutic process, and yet we are human and I strongly believe that our own emotions and experiences can enhance us as therapists. We need to be authentic.

I had so much empathy for Jill and her intense struggles with shame, guilt, and fear. I had also felt those myself in my ED recovery and in my fertility journey (although mine looked somewhat different). I do not believe that I let any of my own pain affect Jill or her process, but it was certainly in the room too (how could it have not been?). We are all human.

I then became pregnant for the third time while working with Jill. When I was several months pregnant I shared my news with her. We processed this together and this became a bonding moment between us. I never told her about my losses as I felt that would have been inappropriate, but knew I needed to process this with her when I got to a point in my pregnancy that was visible to others.

This experience working with Jill and my parallel process was one of the richest therapeutic and personal growth experiences I have had as a clinician, even more so than when I talk with people about my ED (I think this is because my ED has been so far in the past for so long and my fertility struggles have not been). I still feel emotional writing this and thinking about this several years later.

We worked together for a period of time after her baby was born and processed attachment with her daughter, how the ED identity interacted, and so much more. I am grateful to Jill for teaching me so much and helping me grow as a therapist. She also opened my eyes to the intense roller coaster of ups and downs that pregnancy and parenthood can bring. She did so much work on sorting out her values and separating them from her addiction and her ED. She is now a happy and healthy mom to a beautiful 3-year-old!

Jill bonded instantly with her daughter, and she

> was so connected to her and so blissfully happy being with her that none of those feeling came into play. I think the biggest contributing factor [to my bond with my daughter] was breastfeeding. I loved that again my body was able to keep this tiny person alive. I continued to fuel myself and eat healthy/regularly so that my milk supply stayed strong and consistent. I only experienced slight anxiety when it came to being active again. I wanted to run and workout intensely MUCH sooner than the doctor instructed. And I know that desire came directly from my ED reminding me that I wasn't in "good" shape anymore.
>
> Talking a lot about being an example to my daughter was really big [in my recovery]. I never wanted her to struggle the way I did with my ED. Even though she was too young to realize anything I would imagine that she could see me if I was going to binge and purge—that was surprisingly a very strong visual that stopped me several times from going back to ED behaviors. Getting into a swimsuit was very hard as well. I judged myself so much on not being nearly as thin as I was before I had her—a lot of that came from insecurity in my poor relationship with her father as well. When I saw how much she loved being in a floatie in the water it changed my perspective completely. [My daughter] doesn't care what I look like, she only cares about me being with her. It helped tremendously.

All of our experiences are different, yet underneath they can be so very much the same. Shame is the thing that separates us, causes us to isolate and to withhold self-compassion.

When working with pregnant women with an ED in a clinical capacity, I have found it most effective to wear a therapist hat and maintain professional boundaries and ethics, but to truly step into my humanness as well. Whether their therapist is a parent or not, the client needs compassion, non-judgment, and acceptance. They most likely are already experiencing severe criticism from their inner voice (ED voice) and possibly from members of their family and friends. Their therapist might be the one safe person who lets them feel all of their feelings and share their thoughts that they are afraid of saying out loud, such as "I can't do this." Just sitting with them and allowing them the space to have their experience is therapeutic gold.

What Would Mom Say?

Body image is a story told through family systems. As an adolescent's body begins to change during puberty, they turn toward their peers and their parents to understand and "normalize" the experience. Girls grow breasts, hips, and pubic hair, get their periods, and may develop acne. Boys also grow pubic hair, may have acne, and develop a more "manly" physique. Testosterone and estrogen are flowing. This is all in the name of evolution, to help our species adapt and eventually mate to preserve our lineage.

However, it's an awkward time. Hormones are surging for both sexes and bodies grow at a rate that they haven't since they were a baby/toddler. This is a time where body standards become more overt and rampant among preteens and teens and where "fitting in" is one of the life cycle's biggest tasks.

And yet, girls and boys may also learn at that time that their bodies don't quite fit into the "ideal of the day". In fact, this occurs for the vast majority of teenagers as the "body ideal" of the day occurs naturally in only 5% of women and men. Boys may be more lean and lanky than muscular and fit. Girls may be more curvy and have more fat on their bellies and thighs than the standard ideal. All of this is determined by their genetic makeup combined with environmental factors. This is a vulnerable time of identity development among social peers, academic challenges and testing, and learning how to navigate relationships in all capacities.

Teenage girls look to their primary role model as they explore their changing bodies as a way to assess self-acceptance and confidence: their mothers. Mothers are the models for healthy body image and eating behaviors for their kids, especially their daughters. A female role model holds significant power over her daughter's identity development, and a woman's own relationship with her body (including her struggles) will influence this process.

I want to be careful here to step around potential shame triggers for mothers. Kids are made up of part genetics, part environmental influences, and part temperament and personality traits unique to the child. A child can be more or less susceptible to body image and eating issues due to a combination of any of these factors, however no single factor can have complete control of how a child relates to herself and her body. It is an opportunity for a mother or parental figure to pay extra attention to the way that she talks about her own body, how she talks about food and eats, her exercise habits, and to be mindful of the vulnerability quotient of her child.

How Moms Can Support Their Preteen or Teen as Their Bodies Change and Grow (and What Not to Say or Do)

Here are a few strategies for moms to help their children develop a positive body image:

- Talk positively about your own body around your child and try to refrain from negative body talk ("I'm so fat," "I need to lose 5–10 pounds," etc.);
- Similarly, try to talk positively about your daughter's/son's body and refrain from making any negative comments about their weight or shape;
- Normalize food and try not to use good/bad food labels;
- Do not force them to "clean their plate" if they are not hungry;
- Help them identify emotions and body signals;
- Try to eat dinner as a family at least three times per week and make this a bonding and enjoyable event;
- Talk with your child about how bodies change during puberty and empower them to listen to and love their bodies through this (often awkward and uncomfortable) process;
- Know that you are only human and if you feel like you've made a mistake, you can try again;
- Do not put your child on a diet! If they need/want to lose weight, help them reframe that into a positive choice and help them listen to their bodies and needs.

When a woman gets pregnant, the stories of women's pregnancies of her family will most certainly be included in her own experience. From birth plans to how the child is fed once born (breastfeeding or formula?) and sleeping habits (co-sleeping or no? sleep training method?), and don't even get me started on potty-training, there is a never-ending line of advice and pressure (from everywhere!). This life cycle change in a woman's world may bring up old attachment patterns, needs, and wounds that date back to early childhood. Becoming a mother is the most significant identity shift that a woman will ever go through, and she needs her mom to support her. The reality of the type, availability, and dependency of that support may bring up a plethora of emotions from joy to pain to anger.

"In my pregnancy body image story lies my mother's pregnancy body image story," says Kim, 28.

> I tried so hard to not be like her, to not hate my body the way she did while she was pregnant and after I was born. I heard for years how

> awful pregnancy was for her and how "I ruined her body" because it was never the same after I was born. This was painful for me and made me feel like pregnancy is a negative and damaging thing for a woman to experience . . . almost like a "sacrifice."

Penny, 36, shares:

> I am the only daughter/child of a woman who has had a lifelong eating disorder. My mother has long made excuses on why she shouldn't/can't eat. She has made me feel like a glutton for wanting to eat normal food. She is picky. I love everything. My weight has fluctuated over the years, but I only ever hear body positive reinforcement when I was "thin." So when I got pregnant and gained a lot of weight, I felt shame and judgment from her.

Other women look to their moms for an ideal example of how to "bounce back" from pregnancy. Alice, 35, shares:

> My mom has strong ideas about pregnancy and motherhood, almost perfectionistic. Growing up she told me all about her natural labors and her exclusive breastfeeding and when I was pregnant I was terrified of "letting her down" if I didn't follow in her footsteps. This made it quite difficult for me to listen to my own voice and my own body's signals and needs. After giving birth to my son I felt immense pressure from myself (and her internalized voice) to "be like her" and lose the pregnancy weight within six months. I was also dealing with some postpartum anxiety and depression and the whole mix of stress and expectation was so hard.

Clinical Tool: Family Pregnancy and Body Image Genogram

This tool utilizes a genogram to record a family history of how pregnancy was experienced and talked about and the role of body image in this discourse. A genogram, also known as a family diagram, is a pictorial display of a person's family relationships and medical history. It goes beyond a traditional family tree by allowing the user to visualize hereditary patterns and psychological factors that punctuate relationships. It can be used to identify repetitive patterns of behavior and to recognize hereditary tendencies.[11]

This genogram includes: eating disorders/disordered eating, other mental and physical health conditions, pregnancies (including any losses), infertility, and so forth.

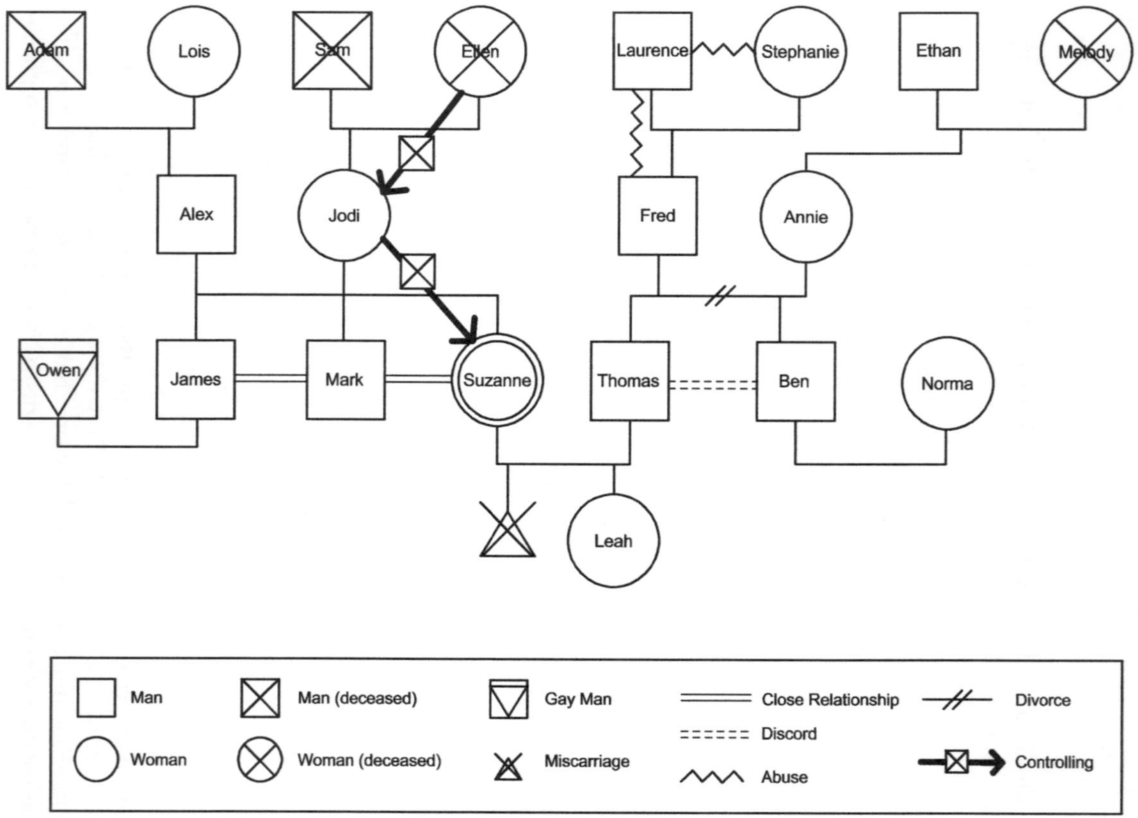

Figure 3.1 An example of a genogram which depicts patterns of emotional, medical, and psychological traits through generations

For consideration: How Did Your Family Pregnancy and Body Image Story Influence Your Own Experience?

Survivor's Guilt and PTSD in Pregnancy

"I never thought I'd be here," says Isabella, 36.

> I've been a part of the online and in-person infertility support groups for over two years. I also am three years into my eating disorder recovery and still go to support groups for those in recovery from EDs as well. I experienced intense survivor's guilt when I found out that we were pregnant—almost like I was leaving behind all of the others. On the happiest day of my life when I felt so much joy, I also felt like I had done something wrong. I know how isolating infertility is, how lonely you can feel in a room of people who are going through the same thing. This is also how I have felt in my eating disorder recovery as it has continued to solidify and become concrete and I know dozens of people (some of them friends) who still struggle every day. I used to look around the room and think: "Who's going to be next? Who will get pregnant and will leave us?" Also, "who is going to recover and I'm not?" I felt such mixed emotions when a group member would get pregnant or would have successes in their ED recovery: both joy for them and also anger. And then that brought up feelings of guilt and of shame.

"Why me and not them? I am now part of the group that the infertility community would call the 'fertile infertiles,'" says Isabella. "I didn't do anything different than they did, I am not any different than those people still suffering. What did I do to deserve being here while they are still struggling back there?"

Survivor's guilt, such as Isabella is feeling, occurs when an individual believes they have done something wrong by surviving a tragic event where others have died or otherwise succumbed. It can manifest across the spectrum, from bittersweet feelings to all-out despair. Most commonly, survivor guilt occurs after a large-scale catastrophe (like a mass shooting or plane crashes), but it can also pop up in unexpected ways, such as with infertility or recovery from a physical or mental illness.[12]

But through counseling and time, Isabella has allowed herself to settle into her pregnancy and to be happy about it. She still has times where she feels guilt and may always do so given her path, but also is able to find some gratitude for her experience because it deepened her recovery and also her self-worth. It is essential for anyone experiencing survivor's guilt of any kind to seek counseling and to work on resolving this in a way that feels most effective for them, as it does not resolve itself on its own. Occasionally, a woman may discover that survivor's guilt she feels at one point in her life is triggered by past guilt or shame narratives in her story—for Isabella, she grew up feeling like having emotions and needs were "wrong" in her family system, and that feeling of being wrong surfaced again now.

Isabella has chosen to take a step back from support groups and from being overly involved in both the infertility and the ED recovery worlds because she experiences some PTSD symptoms such as flashback, increased anxiety, and reactivity when she is too close to those who are going through similar (yet different) issues. She plans to get involved again—if she feels like it—but knows for now she wants to focus on the gratitude and joy she feels for being pregnant—a gift she has yearned for since she was a teenager.

Clinical Tool: Working Through Guilt to Acceptance

Guilt of any shape or form can feel toxic and almost unbearable. Often times it is misplaced and there are more vulnerable or soft feelings underneath. Guilt can feel easier or more comfortable to feel than, say, grief or loss. With guilt, you can direct it toward yourself (albeit unhealthily); with grief and loss there is no parameter, no reasoning.

If you are working with someone experiencing survivor's guilt, try to help them delve deeper and see what lies underneath that the guilt is hiding. Have they let themselves feel the grief and sadness of their time with infertility? Have they truly felt all of the pain and loss of the things their ED took away from them? Try to guide them into these more tender areas and explore them with them compassionately and safely.

Also, hidden beneath survivor guilt is the idea that there's only so much luck to go around and that benefiting from good fortune means that someone else is being deprived of it.[13] Isabella was thinking, "if I get pregnant, does that mean that XXX can/can't get pregnant too?" The mind becomes narrow and rigid when it is stressed out and in pain. It can get into all-or-nothing thinking patterns that feed the shame and guilt. There is not a limited amount of luck or success when it comes to conceiving a child or recovering from an eating disorder. If you do so, that doesn't mean there's any less available for someone else. This concept can be comforting for someone experiencing this and can help them refocus on their own experience and slowly let them sink into the gratitude they have for getting where they are. They deserve it, just as much as anyone else.

Birth Trauma and Eating Disorders

Among the mental health issues that is shrouded in shame and secrecy is post-traumatic stress disorder (PTSD), an anxiety disorder that affects one-third of the people who have experienced a traumatic experience. When we think about PTSD, we most often think about veterans of war or people who have survived a natural disaster or mass shooting. We don't tend focus on the impact of childbirth on a woman's mental health, especially if the birth did not go as planned. Childbirth, a universal experience for all women who have been pregnant, can trigger a previous anxiety disorder to high intensity or initiate a new anxiety disorder. Birth trauma is more common than is openly discussed and can be triggered by unexpected and traumatic experiences during labor, an emergency cesarean section, scary health issues for mom or baby, and an exceptionally long and arduous labor and delivery, among other things. Birth trauma can also be physical, such an injuries to the baby's nervous system during delivery or complications that affect the mother's physical recovery.

Bea, 29, is a mother of two, a boy who is 3 and a girl who is 1. She had no history of an eating disorder prior to her pregnancies, although has struggled with anxiety throughout her life.

> I had no issues getting pregnant; with my son I got pregnant within three months of trying. It was a pretty easy pregnancy, but my labor was horrendous and long. I had to be induced because my son was stuck and was not triggering my body to go into labor. I labored for 36 hours, trying to stay on the positive side, but I was so exhausted that my anxiety spiked. The doctors told me that my baby's heart rate was started to be affected and they needed to do a C-section. I have an intense fear of surgery and wanted to avoid it as much as possible but also wanted my baby to come out. He was so wedged in my uterus that my doctor had to get on top of the table and pull him out. I think that the anesthesia was wearing off because I could feel part of him cutting me up which was awful. I still feel that viscerally and see flashbacks of it. My son was not breathing right away but I was too out of it and in pain to really know what was going on, and no one told me what was going on.
>
> It took them three full minutes to get him breathing. I still remember looking over at him and seeing him not moving and my worst fear almost being a reality. He did eventually start crying and he is okay now but I am traumatized by the entire experience. I don't feel that my doctors really talked to me about my options or gave me options, and I didn't know how to advocate for myself.

Bea began to spiral into anxiety in the weeks and months after she took her son, Max, home. She continued to see flashbacks of him not breathing and feel the doctor cutting her skin. She had panic flowing through her body but didn't know how to help herself. She felt so much shame for not "handling it" the way she "should" and compared herself to other moms. She soon began restricting her eating and cut out dairy, gluten, and sugar, not because of a health concern but because she felt if she lost weight "that was one thing she could feel good about." Bea got pregnant again unintentionally and sooner than she had expected. She wasn't ready. She didn't tell her doctors about her spiral into disordered eating and gained very little weight in her second pregnancy.

Her daughter was born prematurely, and she again felt a spiral of anxiety as she blamed herself for her daughter's health problems due to being born at only 33 weeks. She sought the help of a therapist and dedicated herself to bonding with her children and trying to not let her eating disorder affect her attunement with them.

The intersections of eating disorders and birth trauma are frequent and fascinating and can benefit from further research.

Clinical Tool: Letters to My Baby, Part I

For many women, bonding and connecting with their baby while pregnant is natural. For others, who may have experienced birth trauma in a previous pregnancy, who arrived at pregnancy through an unexpected way either through fertility treatments or having had pregnancy loss(es), or who have pregnancy complications, bonding with their fetus can bring up complex feelings. This tool is a great way for mothers to connect with their child before they are born and to initiate mother-child secure attachment.

Instruct the mother to get a journal or notebook and to write on the cover: "Letters to My Unborn Baby." Inside, the mother writes prompts like "Things I want you to know about me before we meet . . ."; "Promises I make to you . . ."; "Traditions I had when I was a child that I want to pass down to you . . ."; "What I want you to know about your [dad, mother] and me. . . ," "Songs I sang to you while you were in my womb. . .," and so forth. These prompts are intended for mother to talk to her unborn child in a way that is nourishing and future-orienting, to establish comfort and acceptance in the mother's role and that she can look forward to sharing herself and her family with her child.

These can be read aloud in therapy or encouraged to share with her spouse. They also can be kept private for mom to choose to share with her child someday.

Biologically, women's bodies are designed to grow and birth babies. Realistically, there is a wide range of desired and undesired experiences that women go through when considering becoming a parent. A woman may make the decision she does not want to have a child, which she may experience judgment for from societal standards and gender assigned roles. A woman may get pregnant and lose the baby at 7 weeks, or at 28 weeks. She may have an eating disorder and get pregnant and experience a crisis of how to manage this new identity shift. Meanwhile, hormones soar, physical exhaustion endures, and body changes are imminent. This chapter has discussed the wide array of experiences of women in many different situations who become pregnant and who may feel shame or guilt. No matter the circumstances, each woman deserves to know she is worthy and valuable as a human being and as a mother.

Considerations for Therapists

1. How would you support a client who you have countertransference with? Who is going through something that you have experienced, and are you are triggered by it?
2. What are the considerations for assessing a woman's mental health if she has an eating disorder and is pregnant or wants to get pregnant?
3. As important as collaborative care is, what are factors that may prohibit a pregnant mother from disclosing to her medical team that she has an active/recent ED, and how do you as her mental health therapist navigate that situation?

Notes

1. Stone, E. (2013). *A boy I once knew: What a Teacher Learned from Her Student*. New York, NY: Algonquin Books.
2. Tribole, E., & Resch, E. (2012). *Intuitive eating: A revolutionary program that works*. New York: St. Martins Griffin.
3. Tribole, E., & Resch, E. (2012). *Intuitive eating: A revolutionary program that works*. New York: St. Martins Griffin.
4. Tribole, E., & Resch, E. (2012). *Intuitive eating: A revolutionary program that works*. New York: St. Martins Griffin.
5. Fogarty, S., Elmir, R., Hay, P., & Schmied, V. (2018). The experience of women with an eating disorder in the perinatal period: A meta-ethnographic study. *BMC Pregnancy and Childbirth*, *18*(1). https://doi.org/10.1186/s12884-018-1762-9
6. Kimmel, M., Ferguson, E., Zerwas, S., Bulik, C., & Meltzer-Brody, S. (2015). Obstetric and gynecologic problems associated with eating disorders. *International Journal of Eating Disorders*, *49*(3), 260–275. https://doi.org/10.1002/eat.22483
7. Zamora, M.L.C., Bonaechea, B. B., Sanchez, F. G., & Rial, B. R. (2005). Orthorexia nervosa: A new eating disorder? *Actas Esp Psiquiatr 2005;33(1):66–68.*
8. "Fitness" Made Me Infertile. (2018, November 13). Retrieved from www.kiwiandcarrot.com/fitness-made-me-infertile/
9. Postpartum and Antepartum Anxiety. (2019). Retrieved April 24, 2019, from https://www.postpartum.net/learn-more/anxiety-during-pregnancy-postpartum/
10. Easter, A., Treasure, J., & Micali, N. (2011). Fertility and prenatal attitudes towards pregnancy in women with eating disorders: Results from the Avon longitudinal study of parents and children. *BJOG: An International Journal of Obstetrics & Gynaecology*, *118*(12), 1491–1498. https://doi.org/10.1111/j.1471-0528.2011.03077.x
11. Genogram. (2018, December 24). Retrieved December 30, 2018, from https://en.wikipedia.org/wiki/Genogram
12. Hendriksen, E. (2017). Six tips for handling survivor guilt. Retrieved December 30, 2018, from www.psychologytoday.com/us/blog/how-be-yourself/201711/six-tips-handling-survivor-guilt
13. Hendriksen, E. (2017). Six tips for handling survivor guilt. Retrieved December 30, 2018, from www.psychologytoday.com/us/blog/how-be-yourself/201711/six-tips-handling-survivor-guilt

4 Postpartum Attachment and Motherhood

> Birth takes a woman's deepest fears about herself and shows her that she is stronger than they are.
>
> —Unknown

As we continue to look at the journeys of our two primary populations, we enter the chapter of parenthood.

For a recovered woman who experienced fertility issues and ultimately became pregnant, she has a higher chance of enduring comorbid issues like anxiety and depression during her pregnancy and in the perinatal period than a woman who did not incur fertility struggles.[1] In addition, if this woman experienced depression or anxiety previously in her life (as is very common to be an underlying factor to the presence of an ED), the likelihood of her developing PPD or PPA increases as well.

Whether a woman planned to get pregnant, became pregnant by surprise, or somewhere in between, the process of growing a baby in her body and feeling it move inside her is unlike any other experience she will ever have in her life. Giving birth calls upon a woman to trust her body explicitly and unconditionally, as it will take over once labor begins, forcing her to give up control. For a woman who has had or currently has an eating disorder, this may feel like a foreign concept, one wrought in doubt and uncertainty.

Birth also brings a woman to be fully present in her body, to fully immerse herself in it as it embarks on a process that it inherently was built to do, and this fosters opportunity for a restorative process in her mind-body relationship. Kathy, 32, who has a history of an eating disorder and dealt with anxiety over her body changing during her pregnancy, states:

> Feeling the labor pains and not being in control of what my body was doing while I was getting ready to birth my son was the most fascinating process for me. For once I couldn't control it; I just had to surrender. At first I freaked out about what was going to happen next,

> but I trusted my medical team and knew this is what my body was built to do. I let it guide me and it intuitively and gradually moved through the process of birth until I met my son. It was a miracle.

Bringing home and bonding with her baby unveils a mother's deepest capabilities of devotion and surrender, while it also calls upon her most intrinsic coping mechanisms during this significant shift.

Women Who Are Recovered Who Experience Fertility Issues

> In giving birth to our babies, we may find that we give birth to new possibilities within ourselves.
>
> —Myla and Jon Kabat-Zinn

Jennifer, 34, recovered from anorexia and exercise addiction, finally got pregnant naturally after many failed attempts of fertility treatments. She experienced anxiety throughout the first 5 months of her pregnancy, but through the help of counseling, meditation, continuing her anxiety medication, and journaling she was able to manage her anxiety effectively. By the time she delivered, she reported her anxiety to be a 4 on a scale of 1 to 10 (1 being very low; 10 being very high), and felt this was "normal" given her typical anxiety level and the changes coming up in her life.

She delivered a healthy baby boy and immediately felt connected to him. Learning how to help him breastfeed effectively was a struggle at first, but after a few days they got a good latch and he was eating well.

Over time, and through many muddled weeks of little sleep, she began to become overly concerned about his well-being as he grew: Was he eating enough? Is he getting good sleep? What if he gets sick? Am I giving him all that he needs emotionally and physically? These are common thoughts for a new mother to have, especially amid the rigor of sleep deprivation, but for Jennifer she began to see her anxiety intensify. Her baby needed to be held by her almost all hours of the day and had some reflux issues, so Jennifer hardly got any sleep and felt "completely consumed" by her role as a new mother. She felt elated to have her sweet baby boy, but she also felt a loss of her identity and some sadness about that. This in turn increased her feelings of guilt and anxiety. Her husband, while doing the best he could, also struggled with the huge demand of parenthood. He only got one week of paternity leave and developed some symptoms of postpartum depression himself.

Many of these thoughts and feelings are normal for a new parent, but they began to affect Jennifer's own self-care and her relationship with her husband, and she gradually began restricting her food again as a coping mechanism. Jennifer also reports feeling pressure from the media to lose weight and "get her pre-baby body back," and some of the old ED thoughts popped back into her head as she was in a vulnerable state.

Attachment

Mother-child connection, also called attachment, is an essential task in helping the child feel safe and secure to grow into a well-adjusted human. Developing a secure attachment with the baby while it is still in the womb is one of the most crucial psychological tasks during pregnancy and this attachment continues into the postpartum period, helping to determine the mother's ability to adapt to motherhood.[2]

The pregnancy period calls for preparation for a major rearrangement of a mother's life, from reevaluating priorities to relationship changes, financial considerations, new role adaptation, and future planning, among many other things. This requires psychological flexibility and can cause stress for a woman with an active ED or in recovery. EDs are sustained by a rigid, rule-based, closed-off, all-or-nothing mindset, and bringing a new life into the world requires the complete opposite perspective.

If a woman is able to adapt a positive future-based thinking pattern about the impending changes in her life and body and is able to focus on bonding with her fetus, she has a higher likelihood of adapting well to motherhood and forming a secure attachment with her child.

As Jennifer's son began to get older, she adapted more to her new role. But she was also struck by how drastically her life had changed in just a few short months. Finding time to herself seemed almost impossible, and she and her husband felt more disconnected as they tried to stay afloat in the postpartum sea of tasks and jobs.

Jennifer also began to struggle with feelings of guilt and shame, as she did not feel as connected to her son as she felt she "should" (and wished she could). The negative, critical voice in her head made her compare herself to other mothers and created a story about how she was not as "good" as they were at being mothers. This echoed the way the voice talked to her when she was in her eating disorder, just to a slightly different tune. It berated her with mean, irrational thoughts that she kept inside because she was afraid people would think she was crazy or "losing her mind" if she spoke them out loud. She felt horrible and a bit out of control as her food choices became narrower and smaller. To Jennifer, this was one way to try to regain a sense of control and agency in her life—a method that she was very familiar with.

In my interviews, I came across numerous women who shared with me stories similar to Jennifer's. While Jennifer continued to go to counseling and was able to prevent a full relapse of her ED, it is more common than is talked about for women with a history of an ED to "slip" a bit in their recovery when the demands of new parenthood become stressful.

Any major life event can stir up emotion (both positive and negative) and fear, as people who struggle with eating disorders are often resistant to change and new tasks, even if it's a change that is aligned with their values and they truly want it. Situations such as moving away to college, getting one's first job, buying one's first home or moving to a new home, getting married, and certainly getting pregnant and having a baby can trigger inflexible, rigid, fear-based thoughts. These thoughts may live beneath the surface and subconsciously drive the person to use old negative coping mechanisms without them fully being aware. "This is too much, why don't you skip lunch?" or "If you throw up a little bit after dinner you will feel better and tomorrow will be easier to manage," or "I'm the only thing that can help you through this stressful time" are some of the familiar patterns.

What is also remarkable is how a woman's desire and instinct to bond with her baby during pregnancy and postpartum can overrun an ED's attempt at gaining back control of her life. Just as many women fight for recovery because they one day want to have a family and value that so much, this same drive can show up in the pregnancy and postpartum period to fight against ED thinking and behaviors.

Priel and Besser found that mother-baby attachment and bonding serves as a protective factor to psychological distress and disorder during the transition to motherhood and in predicting a mother's ability to adjust to motherhood. If a mother is able to use her resources and find the strength she accumulated during her initial recovery period, she has a high chance of overcoming relapse and attaching securely with her child.[3]

A factor that can lead to more risk of relapse or shame development is the fact that these issues are not openly talked about the way they need to be, although the number of women who endure these struggles is high.

Lori, 29, came to me when she was a new mom to a 3-month-old baby girl. She was just getting back into the workforce after her maternity leave as a sales tech for a wireless company. She reported intense feelings of guilt for "leaving her baby to go to work" and intense feelings of shame for "feeling happy to have a break." She felt stuck in the middle of wanting to go back to work (and needing to go back to work to support her family) because being home with her newborn was so stressful and overwhelming, but also not wanting to miss out on her baby's growth and development while she was working. This is a classic new mom struggle.

Lori had recovered from an eating disorder (classified as a mix of anorexia and bulimia) a few years before she got pregnant and has not had any episodes of lapse since the day she defined herself as "recovered." She wanted to prevent that from ever happening and to work on adjusting to the continual changes in her life as a mom and adapting to her "new normal."

As a mom myself who could very much relate to her struggle, I had to sit and contemplate how to help her. There was no "answer" except self-compassion and self-acceptance, much like in the journey to recovery from an ED.

Next you will find a clinical tool about the power of visualization, which Lori found to be soothing and effective for dealing with her stress. Another intervention that I used with Lori was identifying the different parts of her identity and giving them names and personalities so that they she could understand them and their roles in her reality with less judgment. Lori told me that she felt "lost" and "forgot who she was before the baby." This is common with new parents, whose time and attention is fully demanded by their newborn and baby, and they don't have time or energy to give to parts of them that are underneath. This tool can be helpful in validating a client's experience and helping her to understand her feelings.

Clinical Tool: Identity Web

Lori identified three major parts of herself that are central to her identity: Follower of God, Athlete, and Funny Girl (her words). She and her husband would attend church each week, and Lori grew up being very devoted to God and her religion, which she defined as Christian. She hadn't been able to attend since her baby was born and felt very upset about this. We drew this on paper as a bubble attached to her. In addition, Lori was a runner and had trained for and competed in several half-marathons before she was pregnant. This had been tied in with her ED and had ventured into excessive, but she worked hard at separating the two and reclaiming running as a self-care activity. She ran a bit while newly pregnant but hadn't been running in many months as the exhaustion of pregnancy wore on her. This she felt sad about as well and missed it. We also drew Athlete as a bubble on her identity chart. Finally, Lori missed her Funny Girl, or Silly Self. She remembers going out to play bingo or trivia with friends, or mini-golf or attend concerts. Her sense of humor is one of her favorite qualities about herself and while it's not gone, she feels it has been pushed to the wayside while she cares for her baby and the tries to tackle the amount of work she has to get done. We also drew this on her chart and connected it to her. She drew the bubbles first in the size that she ideally would like them to be, and then in the size and orientation that they currently are. In doing this with clients, you can use as many or few identity bubbles as feels necessary and can continue to add and build on the concept as the client grows.

Lori looked at her identity bubbles and found that those parts are not gone; they might just be smaller while she focuses more intently on her new identity as a Mother. We also processed how to try to integrate these identities together; for example, she is working on planning her baby's baptism, which will tie together her Follower of God identity with her Mother identity. Lori's goal was to try to add more fun into her life, especially with integrating that into her Mother identity. She felt gleeful at thinking about tickling and giggling with her daughter and how that brings her joy.

Over the series of several sessions Lori was able to have a dialogue between different parts of her self, which is a concept drawn from Internal Family Systems (IFS), and gain a new understanding and perspective on her life from a more open and expansive viewpoint.

Clinical Tool: The Power of Visualization

Lori and I worked through a series of visualizations that empowered her to separate herself from her anxiety, guilt, fear, and all of the other uncomfortable feelings she experienced and to remember what (and who) is underneath.

She struggled with feeling "lost" in who she was, which added fuel to the negative thoughts and fears. Shame found a home in this insecure place within her and tried to take up residency.

Here's what you might try with your clients who are like Lori:

> Try to ground yourself in the present moment. Remind your mind that for the duration of this exercise our focus is to be present and that whatever your mind is latched onto from the past and into the future that you will get back to it later. This space is just for you to nurture yourself.
>
> If you feel comfortable, close your eyes and place your feet on the floor. Envision roots coming down through your legs and into the ground, as if you were a tree growing into the floor and spreading. Imagine energy flowing through your body down your legs, through your feet and into the earth in one constant, continual flow.
>
> Tap into your breath. Let it flow with the energy into the earth.
>
> Notice what your body is holding. Where do you feel tension? Pain? Stress? What does it feel like? Describe it—color, texture, temperature, shape.
>
> Don't feel that you need to change anything right now. Our job during the exercise is to observe, notice, describe.
>
> Imagine these negative feelings—the guilt, the fear, the pain [or whatever the client names]—as objects and ask them if they can sit next to you on the couch while we are in this exercise. What does this feel like?
>
> Who is left? What does she have to say? What does she feel? Can you give her a hug?

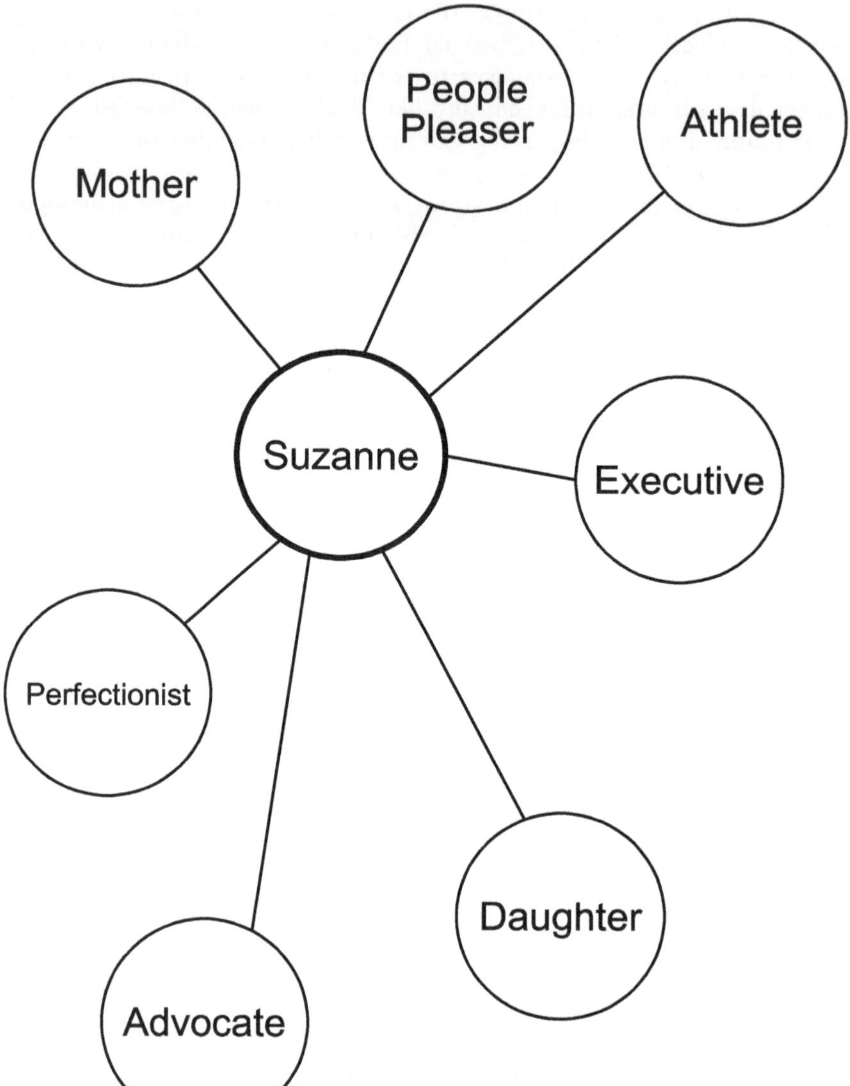

Figure 4.1 An example of identity bubbles, which can be used for any part of the identity

Now bring up in your mind's eye an image of your child (I'm sure this won't be difficult). See her playing. See her laughing. See her crying. Observe her as she feels all of her feelings and experiences.

Can you place her next to you on the couch as well? See her next to you, but not in you anymore. You are a separate but connected being. Can your child give you a hug? As if you are also a child and she is comforting and loving your little child inside.

Give yourself space that it's okay and normal to have all of this on the couch with you. There is nothing "bad" or "wrong" about the feelings sitting to the right of you. For the purpose of this exercise we see that the feelings are separate from who you are but also are connected to you and have much to teach you.

Notice what you are inclined to do. Do you want to move anywhere on the couch? Closer to your child? Away from your child? Away from the feelings? Try not to judge anything, let whatever you feel like doing be okay. What is your child's response to these feelings?

Now bring your child into your lap. Hold her. Feel the energy connecting the two of you.

See if you can accept this experience—all of it, even if it's not perfect or if those feelings still feel super powerful. Try to accept them too.

Breathe in and out. Sit with this experience as long as you would like. Open your eyes when you are ready to come back to the room.

Lori was able to find some relief from her self-criticism with the use of this exercise. She reported feeling more compassion for herself and was able to see that she can be independent and have her own needs while remaining connected to her child at the same time. We used this exercise multiple times over the first few weeks of her adjustment back to work. She noted that she was able to have more power over the negative feelings/thoughts as she practiced this and felt an increased sense of peace and acceptance of her new role.

Postpartum Mood Disorders in Women With EDs

While decades of research has been done on the dangers that eating disorders can pose on a woman's mental and physical health, there is insufficient research about the effects of EDs on a woman's health postpartum.

The postpartum period is a high-risk period for women with EDs, as they are challenged "by the need for a whole new repertoire of coping skills despite having potentially limited internal resources."[4] Motherhood brings a plethora of new social, psychological, and physical stressors, and these coupled with body image concerns due to the physical changes of pregnancy can put women with EDs at a higher risk for developing postpartum mood disorders. In a longitudinal study of women with EDs performed by Franko et al., it was found that nearly 50% of women with active ED symptoms during and after their pregnancies developed postpartum depression (PPD). This is contrasted with women with a history of EDs but no active symptoms, in which 29% of those studied reported

PPD. Both of these populations reported much higher incidences of PPD than in the general population, in which about 10% report PPD. It is also shown in a recent study that more than 90% of women who had a history of an ED reported struggles with new parenthood adjustment up to three months postpartum, compared with 13% of women who had no ED history[5]

I can identify with these statistics on a personal level, and in my work with clients I have felt firsthand the impact of a postpartum mood disorder on a woman's mental and physical health. Anxiety has been something that I have wrestled with throughout my life, and it was an underlying condition to my eating disorder. During periods of major transition (career search, marriage, buying a house, etc.), my anxiety has popped up as I try to grasp the unknown. Even with years of therapy and personal work, I still deal with anxiety regularly.

In many ways, my anxiety during the period of my pregnancy losses and when I was pregnant with my daughter was normal. It makes sense that I would feel nervous and take a breath each day and pray for things to go well as I progressed with my pregnancy with my daughter. As I got further along, to about five or six months pregnant, I felt some relief from the anxiety but it continued to be something I consciously had to distance myself from every day.

After I gave birth to Natalie I was overcome with the joy and gratitude for finally holding this sweet gift in my arms. Simultaneously my anxiety attached itself to my value of being a mother by telling me I "needed to do everything the *right* way" (whatever that means!) and I became overwhelmed with ensuring she was eating enough, sleeping enough, pooping enough, everything enough! Trying to also take care of myself and function in a somewhat effective capacity added new levels of exhaustion and, while normal for any new mom to feel during this massive life transition, for me it at times brought me back to feeling as helpless as I had been against my eating disorder.

I learned to ask for help, and as time went on I grew more confident in my role as a mother (which seems to be an always moving target) and in my daughter's health and resiliency. Anxiety is still something I struggle with and most likely always will, and I think that like for me, any new mom with postpartum anxiety or depression will find that these conditions attach themselves strongly to a value of the mother's.

An example: Hanna, 30, identifies one of her top values as health and wellness. When she gave birth to her daughter, she became overly fixated on the idea that her daughter could not be held or see anyone except her and her husband for the first month of her life due to fears of her daughter getting ill. This extreme representation of her value (health) in reality backfired and caused her to feel more isolated and obsessive about keeping her daughter away from germs so much so that she felt out of control with anxiety. Her heart began beating erratically and she had panicked thoughts and images in her head of her daughter developing a serious illness and needing a long hospital stay. It may be tricky to piece apart what thoughts and behaviors are the result of postpartum anxiety (perhaps it amplifies an underlying worry or feeling) and what is truly a value (such as safety). An essential task for a mother at this stage is to try to identify how she is coping with factors that are new or changing in her life and how she knows when her coping is getting to a place of obsession or extreme, where it is causing suffering to herself and perhaps her baby and partner.

My story aligns in many ways with that of Stephanie, 30. Stephanie struggled to conceive and month after month she felt loss, grief, and disappointment. Her underlying experience of anxiety affected her ability to cope with this very effectively and she began trying to hold on to what she could control. She began meticulously planning her exercise and her diet and tracking her ovulation. Stephanie reports that she has never been diagnosed with an "actual eating disorder," but she watched her mom's own obsession with food and exercise and adopted quite a few of those same behaviors.

When she felt she could not control her fertility, her anxiety worsened. Finally after almost a year of trying, she became pregnant. Her anxiety shifted into "oh my god, how am I going to get ready?" and "can I be a good mother?" Eight weeks after she became pregnant, she and her partner went to the doctor for their first prenatal visit. Stephanie was a mixture of anxiety and excitement; she would finally be able to see her "little bean." As she nervously waited during the exam, the doctor was quiet. "I am so sorry to tell you but I cannot find a heartbeat." Stephanie was in disbelief. She reports feeling "as if the world stopped for a moment."

Following her miscarriage, Stephanie's anxiety worsened further. She could not get out of bed for weeks and blamed herself. She thought "if only I had eaten differently; maybe that would have made a difference." Or, "I exercised too much." She and her partner decided to wait a few months and try again. Now, 2 years later she has a healthy baby boy. Stephanie entered therapy again because "her anxiety is through the roof." She never quite coped with the feelings of loss and anger that she experienced during her fertility struggles and miscarriage. She now reports that she "has nightmares about something happening to her boy and terrible images that flash in front of her eyes." She has never left him with anyone besides her mother or her partner, and even at that, never for longer than 3 hours. In order to cope with this feeling of out-of-control anxiety, Stephanie has begun counting calories and restricting. Her body "is not the way it should be," and she blames herself for this also.

For many women with an eating disorder history, pregnancy can have several effects. For some women, their concern for their unborn child results in a complete cessation of ED symptoms for the duration of their pregnancy; statistics show that 60%–70% of women will go into remission with their eating disorder while they are pregnant. For others it stays the same, gets worse (perhaps due to the lack of control of their body changing and future uncertainty), or changes, as in moving from bingeing and purging to just bingeing.[6] The importance of trying to reduce ED behaviors during pregnancy has been highlighted by the link to poor neonatal and maternal outcomes such as miscarriage, low birth weight, breastfeeding issues and milk supply, preeclampsia, and mortality. Among women whose eating disorder went into remission during pregnancy, up to 75% of them will relapse either partially or back to their pre-pregnancy levels by 18 months postpartum, and it is found that ED behaviors can be more severe postpartum than prior to the pregnancy period.[7]

Research shows that 40% of new mothers, regardless of whether they have a current or past eating disorder, are dissatisfied with their weight and have poor body image after giving birth. Of the women who relapse in their ED postpartum, 80% of them said the top trigger to their ED resurgence was the desire to lost weight due to feeling fat. Many of these women use unhealthy behaviors to lose the weight, which can contribute to feelings of guilt, shame, anxiety, and depression.[8]

In the realm of current eating disorders and postpartum mood disorders, most of the research to date has focus on the connection between BN and PPD. In a retrospective study by Morgan et al.,[9] it was found that of the women who had active BN at the point of conception, one-third developed PPD. Specific behaviors that correlated with the increased risk of PPD included misuse of alcohol at conception, a low body mass index (BMI), increasing bingeing postpartum, and a history of AN, which are all symptoms connected to ED symptomology. Numerous other studies have found connections between current EDs during pregnancy and postpartum mood disorders and have also found a significant link between the severity of PPD and attitudes of perfectionism.[10]

Stephanie felt overwhelmed by the many roles and responsibilities she was trying to juggle and on a daily basis felt as if she "was barely making it through," even though she put pressure on herself to "do everything perfectly." She acknowledged to her partner and to her therapist that she was restricting again and felt shame in that "it made her feel better." Her therapist worked with her to practice self-compassion and to acknowledge that there is a valid reason (although not a healthy one) that her ED resurfaced postpartum. Stephanie began building a community of friends who were also mothers and became more established in her routine with work, taking care of her son, and getting better sleep. By the time her son was 6 months old, Stephanie reports that she "felt more like herself" and while "she'll never be completely the same and is forever changed by her pregnancy experiences," she has more coping tools and has adequately adjusted to her new reality. Stephanie credits "finding a new way to love herself, and falling in love with her son" as cornerstones to her postpartum recovery.

Case Study: Polly

Polly is 38 years old, identifies as polyamorous, bisexual, and agender, and is married to a cisgender man. She works in crisis counseling and says her job is "very stressful and not sustainable full time." She has struggled with depression on and off for as long as she can remember and has a life story of disordered eating related to stress which has resulted in extreme weight gain and loss cycles. She states the disordered eating behaviors have been directly linked to coping with her depression. More recently in her adult life, the behaviors have been qualified as binge eating with periods of dieting and restriction to try to "get healthy" again. Her mother had been in Overeaters Anonymous for many years when she was a child, and Polly feels as if she learned many behaviors from her.

She has had three pregnancies, two of which produced healthy children and one of which ended in a late miscarriage.

> I tend to find myself with an either/or mentality: when I have the focus and energy, I can generally get into healthy patterns; I maintained the weight loss in my 20s for about a decade. But when life becomes stressful I spiral out of control. I do binge eat much of the time, but when I'm in a "healthy" pattern I tend to binge on healthy or low-cal foods, so fruit, cereal, rice cakes, dried seaweed, salads, etc. Pregnancy gave me so much of an excuse to binge, since I had nausea throughout each which was only satiated by food! And depression has compounded my efforts as well, since I eat to self-soothe.

Parenting and her road to get there has brought intense stress for Polly, which she says her bingeing has tried to "help" her cope with.

> My partner and I decided to try to have a child, and it took us about six months for each of our two children. I had a late miscarriage in June 2016. My first child was approximately two at the time. It was physically the most painful experience I've ever had. I was astonished. Emotionally I'm not sure I ever processed it; the physicality was overwhelming.
>
> "Due to my having had my body already stretched out from having weighed much more, and the fact that I know how to get myself into shape when I am motivated, I figured I could handle the change [of my body during pregnancy]. Honestly, I was looking forward to the opportunity to be able to binge eat with an excuse for once! The one thing I didn't factor in was the exhaustion and lack of time for exercise. I figure I can pay more attention to my diet and activity someday, but now is simply not that time. My third pregnancy was so much harder than my first, depression and physical challenges throughout, and so I wasn't really enjoying the increased food intake. I was disappointed with that.

How has her experience with depression and an ED affected her attachment with herself and her children?

> I work my absolute hardest to bond with my kids, but for me it does take some time. I'm definitely closer with my oldest, I'm really not into babies, but once I get to know someone over time then I bond with them. I also have an insecure attachment style myself.
>
> "I don't think my eating disorder has affected bonding that much, to be honest. I do try to encourage my eldest to eat only until his tummy says he's full, and to stop at that point. Upon reflection, we don't have family dinners for a number of reasons, so I may be unknowingly avoiding the issue.

When I checked in with Polly several months later, she told me:

> My daughter is now 13 months and I feel like I've bonded much more with her now. She's a pretty easygoing and cuddly kiddo, so I am finding it easier with her. As the baby became older things generally got easier for me, as I expected, but I don't think she's the cause of the depression. I think it's more closely related to working too many hours, in a room with no windows, than motherhood specifically.
>
> "When I was pregnant, I kept switching OBs until I found someone who would lay off the nutrition talk (as it was triggering and shameful to me). I am working so hard on figuring out healing, but right now I'm in the thick of postnatal sleep deprivation plus full-time work, and I've consciously moved my eating disorder stuff to the background so I can have the energy to focus on the depression and just getting through the day. I only have energy for a wry smile, and I suppose that I'm wagering that by getting to the root of my depression I'll also be getting to the root of the disordered eating.
>
> "I now work in the schools, and I lost about eight pounds over the summer once I finally had time and energy to focus on quality and quantity of eating, and time for more exercise. Eating patterns went back to the old patterns after the school year restarted. I'm trying to incorporate exercise in by walking my son to school most days. There's a part of me that's aghast that I consider a half hour of walking actual exercise, but I also recognize my own bias, and that it's a step in the right direction.
>
> "A potentially interesting development is that I had time to notice, once I finally got a little bit of a break, that food has generally lost its flavor! It's really bizarre. I can tell if something is salty or sweet, and remember what it tasted like. However, it's kind of like the difference between being outside on a vivid day and seeing a grainy picture of that same day. I know what it's supposed to be like, but I can't actually experience it. It hasn't really affected my overeating, though, since eating is more about comfort than flavor.

Polly's story highlights the large spectrum of disordered eating behaviors from restriction, to bingeing, to purging, and everywhere in between that can surface as a "learned" coping mechanism and amid dealing with loss, depression, sleep deprivation, and unfavorable work environments. Polly is a representation of a population of mothers who are in fight or flight mode as they care for their children and put their own needs last. Mothers are heroes and concurrently are at risk of overidentifying with the caregiver role.

Postpartum Attachment in Women Who Have Current EDs

In conjunction with the factors discussed above, a woman with an active ED has higher risk of delivering a preterm and low body weight baby than a woman with no ED symptoms, and due to poor nutrition status she may have difficulty producing the quantity and quality of milk that her baby requires.[11]

The article by Sadeh-Sharvit et al. is groundbreaking in its in-depth look at how an active ED can impact the attachment between mother and toddler. It is one of the few studies on this topic and more research and analysis of this pattern is warranted. This article looked at the trajectory of child development at mealtimes and outside of mealtimes when the mother has an ED—in this case, bulimia. Child adjustment is highly influenced by child-raising practices, patterns, and family culture. In an environment where there is already stress experienced at mealtimes due to the cognitive distortions and maladaptive behaviors associated with an ED, the ability of the child to adapt in a balanced and healthy way is put at risk.[12] The cumulative stress can be very taxing on all family members involved. In a study by Russell, Treasure, and Eisler, it was found that mothers with active anorexia nervosa purposely underfed their children, leading to malnutrition and growth retardation.[13] Additionally, research has shown that up to 50% of mothers with active eating disorders are overconcerned that their child may grow to be overweight, and one study found that mothers are more preoccupied with their daughters' weights than their sons'.[14]

For new mothers who are overly concerned about their own weight and their relationship with food, it has been found that this population is less likely to breastfeed, having more difficulty and less desire to do so than women without eating disorders. Reduced caloric intake, whether due to restriction or purging, may affect milk production and put the baby at risk for malnutrition.[15]

Eating disorder behaviors and symptoms such as food restriction, bingeing, purging, preoccupation with food or exercise, anxiety, and others directly affected the emotional availability of the mother for her child in these case populations. This can have negative consequences for the connection between mother and child and challenge the mother's ability to develop new coping mechanisms to deal with the emergent tasks of motherhood. These studies would benefit from a follow-up several years later as they have predicted the well-being and attachment of the child to its mother with an active ED to be disrupted by the effects of the ED. Numerous studies have shown that when comparing mothers with an active ED with mothers who show no psychopathology, the children of mothers with an ED are at an increased risk of developing ED symptoms and behaviors themselves.[16] As children model their own behavior and self-concept after their primary caregiver (similar to imprinting, such as with baby ducks to their mothers), this is not surprising that the children may feel that ED behaviors are "normal" or may learn that to cope with certain feelings like anxiety, sadness, or anger, they should use food in a way to address or numb them.

Case Study: McKenzie

McKenzie is 25 years old with a son, Mikey, who is 9 months old. She lives with her boyfriend Taylor and stays at home to care for Mikey. McKenzie developed an eating disorder when she was 13 (anorexia nervosa, binge-purge type) and has been to three different treatment centers in her efforts to recover. She has experienced periods of remission and recovery with her ED but struggles to maintain her recovery postpartum. After experiencing a very stressful and "traumatic" birth experience, McKenzie struggled to nurse Mikey and to produce enough milk to satisfy his hunger demands as he grew. As an infant he "cried constantly" and was colicky, and McKenzie began to feel overwhelmed trying to keep up with his demands as Taylor went back to his job as a mechanic just 2 weeks after Mikey was born. McKenzie switched Mikey to formula when he was 3 months old, as her milk production was low due to her own malnutrition and stress.

At 9 months old, Mikey established a healthy weight and began to crawl, babble, and explore the world on his own. He started to eat some solid foods but is "picky," according to his mother. Due to the toll of stress, parenthood, and limited resources and support, McKenzie relapsed into her ED and found herself beginning to overfocus on Mikey's eating habits as a counter-effect to her own preoccupation with food. She wavered between overfeeding him and making him eat more than he needed to (she was unable to listen to his cues or his demands to stop feeding), and she subsequently had anxiety about "how much" he's eating and at times restricted his food when he was hungry. These behaviors were unhealthy attempts for her to soothe her anxiety, which in effect was detrimental to Mikey's emotional and physical growth and development.

McKenzie's anxiety became out of control and she finally asked for help from Mikey's pediatrician. Mikey's doctor related to McKenzie that Mikey was healthy and she did not need to be so preoccupied with his eating schedule and type of food he was consuming. This soothed

McKenzie and she was able to put her anxiety aside in terms of Mikey's care and to follow his doctor's recommendations but her own anxiety and eating disorder spiraled further out of control. McKenzie's mother arrived to stay with her for a few days to help her stabilize and find a better routine with caring for Mikey and for herself.

McKenzie's mother Jan assumed the role of caretaker for both Mikey and McKenzie, while McKenzie became incapacitated by her ED and anxiety and could not complete the tasks of caring for her son. The dynamic between Jan and McKenzie began to echo that of when McKenzie was a child: Jan began to overperform and take control of every aspect of the situation, from Mikey's care, to McKenzie's choices and decisions, to finances, to housecleaning. Taylor began to work more and more to keep up with bills and also to distance himself from the stress of the household. His relationship with Mikey began to become more distant and superficial. His relationship with McKenzie suffered as well, and they argued more regularly as she reverted to a child-like place and became a shadow of her mother.

Here is where we look deeper into attachment between mother and child and how a maternal ED affects a mother's relationship with herself and with her child. In this example we also notice the impact of family systems and relationship dynamics between generations (grandmother-mother-child) on attachment between mother and child and how attachment styles replicate themselves through generational lines.

Attachment in this scope is not looking at parenting styles, discipline, and so forth but on the

> ability to make the child feel safe, secure, and protected. Attachment is where the child uses the primary caregiver as a secure base from which to explore and, when necessary, as a haven of safety and a source of comfort.[17]

Attachment is found to be a significant predictor of a child's future social and emotional outcome.

We notice the delicacy and immediacy of attachment safety that both Mikey and McKenzie are desperate for. Mikey needs this from his own mother, but she is preoccupied with her ED relapse, so his grandmother is taking the place of primary caretaker for him. He looks to Jan now for security, and in doing so he is affected by Jan's own preoccupation with McKenzie, which may have been a factor to McKenzie's ED development when she was barely 13. Clinical assessment shows that McKenzie most likely exhibited fears about gaining weight or losing control much earlier than 13 as a result of Jan's own intense struggle with anxiety and perfectionism.

In a research paper by graduate student Natalie Smitt, *The Experiences of Parents With Eating Disorders*, her in-depth qualitative and quantitative study of parents with EDs found that there was a negative impact on their children including, but not limited to, parentification of the child(ren), social isolation of the child, and emotional absence of the parent. There is little to no research done on the effect of a paternal ED on his children, and this is an area that merits more attention.

Smitt found that these parents worried about and felt guilty about the impact of their ED on their children, how often the ED is their first priority, and that they became preoccupied with trying to hide their ED from their children (especially if the ED consisted of shameful behaviors like bingeing and/or purging). An interesting finding of her research was that many parents she interviewed cited challenges with finding adequate and effective treatment as a parent with an ED. This might be due to availability of treatment centers, financial resources, and finding childcare while the mother attends treatment.[18]

Another factor that may prevent a mother from addressing her ED and seeking help is fear of losing custody of her child(ren). McKenzie was resistant to going back to treatment another time, even though her family was encouraging it, out of fear of losing custody of Mikey to Taylor or to her mother. She minimized and tried to hide her ED behaviors, which consisted of purging after eating (no episodes of bingeing), and the stress of attempting to keep the ED covert while maintaining it and her other responsibilities caused her to further decompensate in her functioning ability.

A study by Dipple et al. in 2002 found that 68% of mothers with mental illness of any kind were permanently separated from at least one of their children before their child was 18. This staggering and pathologizing statistic validates McKenzie's fears of losing custody of Mikey and being present in his life. Mental illness of any kind can be stigmatized, leading to a family potentially being broken up and losing those connections that are so desperately wanted and needed. Of mothers who do go to treatment to try to recover from their mental illness, they may minimize or avoid talking about their parenting responsibilities out of shame of not being a "good enough" mother and wanting to appear to be functioning well.[19]

Societal prejudices about mental illness may also convince a mother that she is innately "inadequate" at parenting and that any problem that her child has, even if it's a normal developmental concern, is her fault. Additionally, a mother's competence may be affected by her mental disorder and she may feel guilt over the effect that the disorder is having on her children. This can interfere with her making and holding appropriate boundaries with her children or being lax with their discipline. Further research is warranted on the specific impact that a maternal eating disorder has on the parent-child relationship and if it is correlated with effects of other mental illnesses.

McKenzie felt this weight on her and began to retreat further and further inside of herself, internalizing the stigma of being a mother with an eating disorder and feeling like she was "failing" the societal standards of what a mother should be. Her ED mindset told her in very rigid and catastrophic thought patterns: "You're a terrible mother. You deserve to wither away because you can't do the one thing you're supposed to do right now: take care of your son." "He's better off with your mother." "You're messing him up beyond repair." "Other mothers have it all together and are not as messed up as you are." Consequently, her actions began to correlate with her negative self-concept and she withdrew from Mikey while in her ED, but also vacillated and became overconcerned with his feeding, sleep, care, and so forth at times when her anxiety was peaked.

Research verifies that a social network and community for new parents is a strong buffer for developing postpartum mood disorders and can help manage their symptoms in the case they do develop.[20] Parent community can prevent isolation and foster a sense of belonging and confidence in figuring out how to adapt to the massive life changes that any new parent endures. Parents such as McKenzie who are struggling with a mental illness of some type may feel stigmatized and ashamed of their condition and withdraw from social support opportunities, putting them at further risk for maladaptive coping mechanisms.

McKenzie is currently assessing her options for treatment and is considering entering an intensive outpatient program at a local treatment center. She has recognized the severity of her eating disorder and that she deserves a better life than the one she currently has. While she is unwavering in her commitment to wanting to be there for Mikey, McKenzie said, "I need to do treatment and recover for myself. I deserve that. I can't do it just for him."

Parent-Child Attachment in Recovery

Interestingly, research has found no negative effects from an eating disorder on the mother-child relationship if the mother has been in sustained recovery for several years. In healing effectively from her own eating disorder, she is creating a safe and secure relationship with herself that lays the groundwork for a secure attachment with other important relationships (partner, child, etc.). If a woman has prenatal anxiety or depression, these may have a higher likelihood of emerging during the perinatal period if a woman has an eating disorder, which can impact attachment with the child.

Genna, 37, a parent to a 5-year-old son and pregnant with her second child (she had a miscarriage in between her pregnancies), had a severe eating disorder (a mixture of bulimia and restriction) beginning when she was 11. Through intense treatment and family support, she has been in recovery since 2006. She told me about her experience becoming a new parent from the perspective of someone in recovery from an ED:

> I was very fortunate to not have experienced any postpartum mood disorders with my first. My ED past has made me a better mother, and overall person. Sitting with uncomfortable feelings has been the primary tool for my recovery. I had such a hard time tolerating uncomfortable feelings because I was raised in an environment where feelings were not discussed, or even tolerated. If you have a bad feeling—you toughen up and deal with it. There was no discussion of feelings, they were something to get over. My parents did not have any patience for crying, disappointment, anxiousness, hurt. And once I moved out, became an independent "adult" with lots of feelings, I had no idea how to deal with them, or even accept them.
>
> So with my son, we embrace all the feelings—good and bad. My history with my ED and family history led me to research and utilize respectful/gentle parenting. I have gotten my husband on board with the same. Parenting my son has been such a joy and he is growing to be such a sweet, kind and empathetic kid.
>
> Without my history with my ED and my recovery, I don't know that I would parent consciously. But my ED gave me motivation to want to do things differently for my children. I look at how my childhood lead me to my ED and when I raise my children, I want to raise them to be functional, happy, successful adults vs. "obedient children." I parent with an end goal in sight and try to provide my son with the tools that he will be able to use into adulthood. Without my ED, I don't know that I would even have the perspective to parent any differently.

For others, the experience of parenting can trigger a postpartum mood disorder (PPMD) after the birth of one of their children but not others. Lia, 36, a parent to three children, struggled with anxiety and bulimia for 7 years in high school and college. She is now fully recovered and reflects on her attachment and security in her parent role:

> I did not experience PPMD with my first two, a fact that I attributed to longer than usual maternity leaves. (I stayed home for six months with my daughter and just over four months with my son.) With my third, though, I have absolutely experienced PPMD, most often manifesting as anxiety, a massive feeling of overwhelm, and anger. With all of my babies, though, I can honestly say that I have felt unsteady in the postpartum period. My body has felt foreign, and my eating more chaotic. As is normal in breastfeeding mothers,

> I've needed a lot of carbs, which eating disorders taught me to question and even early recovery taught me to incorporate mindfully. But postpartum and breastfeeding necessitated that I be mindful of other things, and my hunger and carb cravings would often sneak up on me and, if I'm honest, scare me a bit. This time around, I won't say I'm any more mindful, but I will say I'm gentler with myself. This is a season, and my body knows what it's doing, even if it feels a little unhinged to me.

Clinical Tool: Letters to My Baby, Part II

Part II of the tool from Chapter 3, this exercise helps mothers connect with their child in a way that they can feel safe and secure. This can be done with mothers who completed letters to their unborn child, or this can be a separate exercise completely. Mothers who experience postpartum anxiety or depression may feel guilt or sadness about their mental illness affecting the attachment they have with their child(ren). Here, a mother can write about her experience with motherhood and with mental illness from a less internalized or personalized perspective.

She can take out her journal and write letters: "What I wish I could say to you that I struggle to say . . ."; "What you mean to me . . ."; "What I love about being a mother to you . . ."; "You make me smile when . . ."; "What I want you to know about mom's feelings . . ."; "When I was your age, I . . ." and so forth. These are written to her child (newborn to age 10) and stored in a box. She can choose to share them with her child when they are older, or keep them for herself. This can help take away the stigma and self-judgment that she may have about her parenting and allow forgiveness and acceptance.

As a reminder, attachment is not the same as bonding, which is a common misconception made by clinical professionals and non-clinicians alike. It is not associated with how a child is fed, how they are taught or disciplined. Rather, attachment is defined as "where the child uses the primary caregiver as a secure base from which to explore and a safe haven and a source of comfort."[21] There are three forms of organized attachment: secure, avoidant and resistant, and one disorganized type.

In my interviews, I found a common theme of parenting styles associated with "helicoptering," as one woman described it. In clinical terms, this organized attachment style would be described as anxious-preoccupied in women who have an active or recent eating disorder. For women who are still active in some ED behaviors and cognitions, the most common attachment style with their child is insecure-dismissing, as was the case with McKenzie. The type of attachment that an infant develops with their caregiver is determined by the caregiver's response to the infant when the infant's attachment system is "activated," meaning their feelings of safety and security are threatened, such as when he/she is physically ill or are emotionally upset (e.g., frightened).

Attachment styles such as avoidant or resistant are classified as "organized" because the child has adapted to their caregiver's way of responding to them and have learned how to find ways of feeling safe even if in dysfunctional ways.

Eating disorders pose a complexity in the fabric of a new mother's psychological, physical, and emotional adjustment to a new life stage. Even without the presence of an eating disorder, new parenthood initiates a "normal life crisis" that requires strong coping skills as parents learn how to feed and care for an infant—along with themselves. While there can be numerous risks to baby and mother if an eating disorder is present in the perinatal period, if a mother is in full recovery or taking steps to do so, she can develop a secure attachment with her child, lower her risks of developing a PPMD, and show signs of resiliency in many life challenges. Therapists working with mothers in this population are encouraged to triage with her care team and help the mother and her partner find many resources to support recovery as a new parent.

Considerations for Therapists

1. How would you depict and define the attachment style your client, who is a new mother with an active eating disorder, has with her child(ren)? What would you look for?
2. What type of attachment style do you have with your primary caregivers? How has this evolved in your lifetime and with your own children, if you have any?
3. What resources are called for (assessment tools, screenings, etc.) in supporting the population of mothers with past or active eating disorders, especially in helping to identify risk factors for developing PPD or PPA?

Notes

1. Astrachan-Fletcher, E., Veldhuis, C., Lively, N., Fowler, C., & Marcks, B. (2008). The reciprocal effects of eating disorders and the postpartum period: A review of the literature and recommendations for clinical care. *Journal of Women's Health*, *17*(2), 227–239. https://doi.org/10.1089/jwh.2007.0550
2. Lai, B.P., & Tang, C.S. (2008). The negative impact of maternal bulimic symptoms on parenting behavior. *Journal of Psychosomatic Research*, *65*(2), 181–189. https://doi.org/10.1016/j.jpsychores.2008.04.003
3. Priel, B., & Besser, A. (2000). Adult attachment styles, early relationships, antenatal attachment, and perceptions of infant temperament: A study of first-time mothers. *Personal Relationships*, *7*(3), 291–310. https://doi.org/10.1111/j.1475-6811.2000.tb00018.x
4. Astrachan-Fletcher, E., Veldhuis, C., Lively, N., Fowler, C., & Marcks, B. (2008). The reciprocal effects of eating disorders and the postpartum period: A review of the literature and recommendations for clinical care. *Journal of Women's Health*, *17*(2), 227–239. https://doi.org/10.1089/jwh.2007.0550

5. Koubaa, S., Hällström, T., & Hirschberg, A. L. (2008). Early maternal adjustment in women with eating disorders. *International Journal of Eating Disorders, 41*(5), 405–410. https://doi.org/10.1002/eat.20521
6. Fogarty, S., Elmir, R., Hay, P., & Schmied, V. (2018). The experience of women with an eating disorder in the perinatal period: A meta-ethnographic study. *BMC Pregnancy and Childbirth, 18*(1). https://doi.org/10.1186/s12884-018-1762-9
7. Lacey, J.H., Smith, G. (1987). Bulimia nervosa: The impact of pregnancy on mother and baby. *British Journal of Psychiatry, 150*, 777.
8. Lemberg R, Phillips J. (1989). The impact of pregnancy on anorexia and bulimia nervosa. *International Journal of Eating Disorders, 8*, 285.
9. Morgan, J.F., Lacey, J.H., Sedgwick, P.M. (1999). Impact of pregnancy on bulimia nervosa. *British Journal of Psychiatry, 174*, 135.
10. Astrachan-Fletcher, E., Veldhuis, C., Lively, N., Fowler, C., & Marcks, B. (2008). The reciprocal effects of eating disorders and the postpartum period: A review of the literature and recommendations for clinical care. *Journal of Women's Health, 17*(2), 227–239. https://doi.org/10.1089/jwh.2007.0550
11. Stewart, D.E., Raskin, J., Garfinkel, P.E., MacDonald, O.L., Robinson, G.E. (1987). Anorexia nervosa, bulimia, and pregnancy. *American Journal of Obstetrics and Gynecology, 157*, 1194.
12. Sadeh-Sharvit, S., Levy-Shiff, R., Arnow, K.D., & Lock, J.D. (2016). The interactions of mothers with eating disorders with their toddlers: Identifying broader risk factors. *Attachment & Human Development, 18*(4), 418–428. https://doi.org/10.1080/14616734.2016.1164201
13. Russell, G.F., Treasure, J., & Eisler, I. (1998). Mothers with anorexia nervosa who underfeed their children: Their recognition and management. *Psychological Medicine, 28*(1), 93–108. https://doi.org/10.1017/s003329179700603x
14. Agras, S., Hammer, L., & McNicholas, F. (1999). A prospective study of the influence of eating-disordered mothers on their children. *International Journal of Eating Disorders, 25*, 253.
15. Lacey, J.H., Smith, G. (1987). Bulimia nervosa: The impact of pregnancy on mother and baby. *British Journal of Psychiatry, 150*, 777.
16. Reba-Harrelson, L., Holle, A.V., Hamer, R.M., Torgersen, L., Reichborn-Kjennerud, T., & Bulik, C.M. (2010). Patterns of maternal feeding and child eating associated with eating disorders in the Norwegian Mother and Child Cohort Study (MoBa). *Eating Behaviors, 11*(1), 54–61. https://doi.org/10.1016/j.eatbeh.2009.09.004
17. Benoit, D. (2004). Infant-parent attachment: Definition, types, antecedents, measurement and outcome. *Paediatrics & Child Health, 9*(8), 541–545. https://doi.org/10.1093/pch/9.8.541
18. Smitt, N. (2012). *The experiences of parents with an eating disorder*. Australia: Monash University.
19. Dipple, H., Smith, S., Andrews, H., & Evans, B. (2002). The experience of motherhood in women with severe and enduring mental illness. *Social Psychiatry and Psychiatric Epidemiology, 37*, 336–340. https://doi.org/10.1007/s00127-002-0559-2.
20. Micali, N., Simonoff, E., & Treasure, J. (2011). Pregnancy and post-partum depression and anxiety in a longitudinal general population cohort: The effect of eating disorders and past depression. *Journal of Affective Disorders, 131*(1–3), 150–157. https://doi.org/10.1016/j.jad.2010.09.034
21. Benoit, D. (2004). Infant-parent attachment: Definition, types, antecedents, measurement and outcome. *Paediatrics & Child Health, 9*(8), 541–545. https://doi.org/10.1093/pch/9.8.541

5 Shame and Perfectionism

Brené Brown, a research professor at the University of Houston who has spent the past two decades studying courage, vulnerability, shame, and empathy calls shame "the swamp land of the soul." It is "the intensely painful feeling or experience of believing that we are flawed and therefore unworthy of love and belonging—something we've experienced, done, or failed to do makes us unworthy of connection."

"I think shame is much more likely to be the source of destructive, hurtful behavior than the solution or cure. I think the fear of disconnection can make us dangerous," she says.[1]

In this book we have met numerous women who struggle with feeling not good enough to be a mother; who desire desperately to have a child but cannot; who binge and purge or starve themselves while they are pregnant with their child and cannot stop no matter how desperately they want to; whose vision of motherhood has not panned out the way they'd hoped for and dreamed about.

These experiences of pain, lack of control, and loss can set the scene for shame and guilt to seep in. They may entertain thoughts of "did I do this to myself?" "It's my fault . . . my eating disorder is the reason I cannot have a child." "Am I harming my child with my behaviors?" "What if I can't be a good enough mom?" and "I don't know if I want this child," among hundreds and hundreds of other intrusive thoughts. Thoughts that live in the deep depths of the subconscious and speak to their greatest fears. Thoughts that seep to the surface into consciousness and deepen the shame of their experience.

Eating disorders thrive in shame and secrecy; it is their bread and butter. This chapter will focus on the lived experiences of the two highlighted populations and bringing the shame they may have felt into light. It will also look at tools that therapists and support systems can use to try to decrease shame and navigate the woman toward self-acceptance. What I would hope for women to hear that fall into any of these categories is: *your worth is not defined by the status of your womb.*

How Does Perfectionism Feed Shame?

And what about perfectionism? What is its relationship to shame? How do they go hand and hand in sustaining an eating disorder and preventing a woman from living the value-based life that she desperately, truly wants to live?

The dictionary describes perfectionism as "a personality trait characterized by a person's striving for flawlessness and setting high performance standards, accompanied by critical self-evaluations and concerns regarding others' evaluations." It is also characterized by "refusal to accept any standard short of perfection."[2] The definition of perfectionism has been debated by researchers as of late, and its role in psychopathology such as depression, anxiety, and eating disorders is complicated. Kenneth Rice, PhD and his colleagues find it problematic that some call perfectionism "adaptive," meaning that it serves a specific function to help an organism's survival. He sets apart having high standards from the condition of perfectionism, which runs deeper into one's self-concept and can cause "belief that others will value you only if you are perfect." High standards might be adaptive in one situation but not another, or for certain people but not others, he says.[3]

Psychologist Gordon Flett studies "socially prescribed perfectionism," which has an element of pressure combined with feelings of helplessness and hopelessness. Socially prescribed perfectionists, he notes, tend to feel that "the better I do, the better I'm expected to do."[4] Women who desire to be mothers or who are mothers are vulnerable to socially prescribed perfectionism and are at risk for feeling they need to be a "perfect mother" as society prescribes: this may involve tasks such as giving birth ("make sure it's unmedicated and a water birth"), feeding their child ("breastfeeding is natural and best"), sleep ("don't let them cry it out!"), discipline ("don't do time outs, do time ins"), and more; the expectations are limitless, stressful, and often contradictory. For a sleep-deprived, anxious new mother, this can be dangerous.

This endless cycle of perfectionistic narratives of "not good enough" or "never enough" can increase one's vulnerability to developing or relapsing on an eating disorder (or other mental health issues), which is sustained on a rigid, all-or-nothing mindset and also is derived from a socially prescribed standard. Pregnant and new mothers feel immense pressure to maintain a "healthy ideal" and stay fit (thin) during pregnancy and postpartum. If one fits the "social ideal"—in body shape or size (the "thin ideal"), in social class, in skin color and ethnicity, in sexual orientation, etc.—then one is "good enough." If you deviate from that, like the vast majority of the world's population does naturally, you are at risk for judgment and stigma from those that prescribe to the social ideal, feeding shame and the perfectionist mindset. This is the petri dish for an eating disorder or other maladaptive coping strategies.

Perfectionism isn't a behavior; it's a way of thinking about yourself, says Andrew Hill, a researcher. It is developed from a combination of genetics, temperament, personality type, and life experiences—basically how a person has adapted to their surroundings and biological makeup. For some, this could be having high standards for themselves but not thinking negatively of themselves if they do not measure up. This is called adaptive perfectionism, whose validity is up for debate. Researchers argue that trying to reach a certain goal is not perfectionism, it is conscientiousness—a natural instinct to grow and perform. Maladaptive perfectionism is when a person internalizes their ability to achieve a certain standard and judges herself based on her ability to "be perfect." It's that critical inner voice, which is not present or not as self-focused in a person who strives to achieve a goal and works hard at it. Take an example of the student who studies hard to get a certain grade on an exam, but falls short of what she hoped to get. She tells herself: "I'm disappointed, but it's okay; I'm still a good person overall." In contrast a perfectionist might tell herself: "I'm a failure. I'm not good enough."[5] This is toxic.

Unfortunately, modern society celebrates maladaptive perfectionism and reinforces it through marketing, television, and social media. You see this in commercials for clothing, makeup, and accessories, targeted at girls as young as 8 and featuring actors who are not necessarily realistic. For many vulnerable adolescents and teenagers (girls and boys), they may think: "oh, if I buy this product and lose weight, then maybe I can be as happy and beautiful as the person in that commercial." Statistics back this up:

- Approximately 7 in 10 women and girls report a decline in body confidence and increase in beauty and appearance anxiety, which they say is driven by the pressure for perfection from media and advertising's unrealistic standard of beauty.
- Almost 8 in 10 girls (79%) and even more women (85%) admit to opting out of important events in their lives when they don't feel they look their best.
- Nine out of 10 women say they will actually not eat and risk putting their health at stake when they feel bad about their body image. And 7 in 10 girls said they're more likely to be less assertive in their decisions when they're feeling insecure.
- To counteract these unreal messages, a majority of women and girls around the globe are challenging media to portray more diverse physical appearances, age, race, body shapes, and sizes.[6]

While there has been some movement to change the dialogue in marketing and make it more inclusive (see the recent Dove commercials, for example), our society still has a long way to go to try to unravel the negative self-esteem messaging that we are sold.

Perfectionism starts young: one woman I interviewed described remembering feeling intense feelings of disappointment, even shame, when she was maybe six years old and messed up a drawing she was coloring. She destroyed it right away and had thoughts like "you're so stupid" and "you're messed up" for days afterwards. This personality trait can develop early, especially if a girl grows up in a family system that portrays and exacerbates perfectionism. Perfectionism in adolescents is rapidly increasing, spanning into adulthood and bringing along with it a plethora of other mental health issues.

Thomas Curan and Andrew Hill's recent groundbreaking meta-analysis of perfectionism over generations from 1989–2016 found significant increases in rates of perfectionism in the United Kingdom, the United States, and Canada. "As many as two in five kids and adolescents are perfectionists," says Katie Rasmussen, who researches child development and perfectionism at West Virginia University. "We're starting to talk about how it's heading toward an epidemic and public health issue." The rise in perfectionism does not mean that we are getting more accomplished—quite the opposite. We are getting more depressed, more stressed out, and undermining our own potential and self-worth at the hands of perfectionism. It is quite self-defeating and is steeped in irony: making and admitting mistakes is a necessary part of growing and learning and being human. It also makes you better at your career and relationships and life in general. By avoiding mistakes at any cost, a perfectionist can, ironically, make it harder to reach their own lofty goals.[7]

Given this research, it comes as no surprise that perfectionism is strongly linked to anxiety and eating disorders, as an eating disorder can develop as a method to adapt to modern society's standards and cope with the critical inner voice and anxiety that consumes them.

Here's where I need to do some self-disclosure. I am an admittedly "recovering perfectionist" myself, having had perfectionistic tendencies for as long as I can remember. I am certain that they contributed to the development of my eating disorder and still maintain some of my anxiety to this day. Writing this book has been the biggest challenge to my perfectionism that I have ever encountered (well, maybe next to my recovery from my ED) and has resulted in more than a few instances of panic and anxiety-ridden dreams. What sets me apart from 20-year-old me is that I realize the pressure that I am putting on myself is not realistic and is actually much more damaging than productive. This does not mean it's easy to "turn off" that drill sergeant in my head, but through the process of writing I am learning that my voice is valid just as it is. I don't need to be "perfect" to write a valuable, intelligent, and accessible book. I just need to be me and to appreciate that person. This is my lifelong mission and I am dedicated to helping prevent my daughter from suffering from perfectionism like I have. You may have a perfectionism demon in your head as well, and if you do, just know that you can push past it and do great things without listening to it.

When Recovery Matters More Than Being Perfect

For women who desire to get pregnant and who are in recovery from an eating disorder, dedicating themselves so forcefully to recovery may have been in part because they one day wanted to be healthy enough (in mind and body) to carry their own child and become a parent. They work tirelessly to challenge those perfectionistic triggers and to connect with the values that they most naturally embody: to be a parent and nurture a new life. I don't think that anyone is truly perfect at this (ironically) but can make significant strides through therapy and self-reflection and see that they are a "good enough" parent, woman, partner, or member of society just as they are.

In my experience working with clients and as a parent myself, I find that arriving at a middle ground and embracing the "gray" is essential to a healthy and sustained recovery. However, when women who have perfectionism come up against struggles with fertility or sustaining a pregnancy that appear out of their control, they may once again be vulnerable to perfectionistic all-or-nothing thinking, such as "the harder I try, the more I fail" or "I need to become the healthiest I can be to be able to get pregnant." The evil stepsister of perfectionism—shame—can come in when despite all of their efforts they still struggle to have the family or role of parent that they once envisioned for themselves.

Hewitt, Flett, and their colleagues have found a connection between self-oriented perfectionism (an internally motivated desire to be perfect) and anorexia nervosa. They see perfectionism as a risk factor to anorexia, not a disorder in and of itself, and the condition will not directly correlate with the development of an ED. When stress is low, self-oriented perfectionists tend to do well, but when things go wrong—or not as expected—they are more at risk to develop depression, anxiety, suicidality, and eating disorders.[8]

In my own story, my value of family was a significant part of my commitment to recovery—someday I wanted to have a career that was meaningful to me, a marriage, and a family, and I could not fathom doing those things with my ED being so strong. I had to make a choice, and at that point it needed to be black-or-white decision-making: ED or life.

What is striking to me about this point in my recovery is that so much of recovery beforehand was gray, and the discomfort of trying to live in the gray was meaningful yet painful. Here was a clear choice: if I wanted to live the life I dreamed of, I could not use any ED behaviors or follow any ED thoughts (even though they might still pop up occasionally). I needed to put my inner perfectionist in a box where she could not have so much negative influence on my decisions or self-concept. I needed to feel my pain and all of my emotions instead of mask them with an eating disorder. I deserved to feel worthy as a human being without looking a certain way or prescribing to an unattainable social ideal.

Yet when we started trying to conceive and began down a road of loss and pain, thoughts popped into my head: "Did I do this? Is it my fault that my body can't sustain a pregnancy? Is it because of my ED?" Shame seeped in. An excruciating pain that I had never experienced before. And deep, deep anger at my ED for robbing me of my life's happiness, even so many years later. My perfectionistic thinking reemerged during this time of intense stress, and I felt that there was not enough I could do or try to regain a sense of control over the situation.

What lies underneath the layer of perfectionism—the vulnerable part that the inner perfectionist is perhaps trying to "protect"—is one's strong desire to be accepted and cared for by oneself and by others for being who they are. This relates to attachment theory, which describes human beings' innate need to feel loved and safe and secure, and if there is a disruption in this bond with a caregiver then maladaptive coping mechanisms are developed as a protective factor. If a parent regularly criticizes her daughter for her weight, shape, or overall appearance, this can become internalized by the child as "I am not good enough as I am" and "It's not safe here to be who I am," and she may subconsciously utilize disordered eating or self-harm behaviors in order to compensate for this painful wound.

Children of mothers who are overly concerned about their weight are at increased risk for modeling their mother's unhealthy attitudes and behaviors,[9] and up to 40% of overweight girls and 37% of overweight boys are teased about their weight by peers or family members. Weight teasing predicts weight gain, binge eating, and extreme weight control measures including disordered eating, laxative abuse, and poor self-esteem.[10]

Sasha, 37, a mother of two young girls ages 5 and 7, struggled with bulimia from ages 14 to 25, which was a deep source of shame for her. She feels it developed due to a mixture of "intense school and parental pressure and my own harsh self taskmaster." Her mother had struggled with her own weight and perhaps an unacknowledged eating disorder for her entire life, and Sasha remembers her

> always being on a diet: Atkins, the grapefruit diet, she'd try them all. There would also be days where she would not eat anything. She was very judgmental towards people who gained weight, including her kids. I feel fairly certain this influenced my attitudes toward weight that contributed to developing an ED. My parents also treated it like a fairly inconvenient secret—both were aware of my eating disorder, but only half-heartedly recommended help before sending me off to college across the country. I don't know if it was shame or apathy, but when I think back I'm shocked that they let me take that risk to my health (bulimia plus collegiate distance running) without more intervention. That obviously wasn't my own personal motherhood experience, but becoming a mother has definitely helped me realize that some of these things were very damaging to me.

In her own motherhood experience, she has diligently tried to repair and rewrite the narrative of food and weight with her daughters, letting them eat what they want without shame. Sasha struggled with a couple of relapses after her initial recovery period and was deeply ashamed of this. She told no one about her eating disorder past, and when she was doing prenatal counseling with her doctor, she was too embarrassed to bring it up. Her doctor did not ask her about it either, so it was not discussed. Sasha's perfectionist mindset still told her that it was her fault that she had developed an eating disorder and that she would never attain the "perfect" ideal of motherhood—a leftover wound from her own childhood. Sasha knows her daughters may be vulnerable to EDs due to her own and her family's history, but commits herself to be conscious about how she talks to them and about her own body. She may slip up and fall into old patterns mimicking her own mother's style, but she is learning to recognize this and offer herself compassion instead of judgment. In this way, she is setting the stage for secure attachment that she never got, and helping her daughters develop a more affirming and less rigid inner voice of their own.

In situations where shame and inner criticism are not intervened with and continue to grow and feed off one another, more maladaptive coping mechanisms like addiction, avoidance, and deeper ED issues are at risk of developing. Relief comes in the form of acceptance. Self-acceptance and the acceptance of where one is on their journey in life can directly challenge the ED and perfectionistic mindset. But how does one achieve this if it feels far from natural?

For many, this entails acceptance of a radical nature: radical acceptance means completely and totally accepting something from the depths of your soul, with your heart and your mind. You stop fighting reality. When you stop fighting, you suffer less.[11] Perhaps this means that they will not be able to have children; that their pregnancy loss is real and cannot be avoided or denied; that they are not further along in their recovery as they might have hoped; that their eating disorder gets in between the connection she has with her child. Once acceptance is found, no matter how undesirable or unintended it might be, moving forward to the next step of healing is possible.

In my research I interviewed one woman with a unique experience with infertility. Breanna, now 28 and single,

> flirted with disordered eating my whole life, but once I got to grad school at age 22 anorexia nervosa had completely taken over. I had done extreme dieting and restricting/binging phases through all of high school and college, but always maintained my weight. When I was in grad school in a fast pace, high stakes nursing program that left no room for error I found myself striving for perfection. It was also around this time I was told my endometriosis was severe and

> I would likely never have children. Since I had dysfunctional uterine bleeding and endometriosis both of which exacerbated the other, I was told I could not have children before I even got the chance to encounter a realistic opportunity. After 2 more years of trying to hold onto some hope I realized all the doctors were right and at 26 I got a hysterectomy.

Breanna's eating disorder was both a coping mechanism for the reality of her fertility health and also the thing that robbed her of it.

> My anorexia took over my life around the time I was told I could not have children. It was devastating, I had already spent two years trying to treat the abnormal uterine bleeding without knowing I was feeding the endometriosis I had yet to be diagnosed with. I kept trying for three more years to control the bleeding in hopes the doctors were wrong. I started trying to eat a low inflammatory diet to try and control the endometriosis, then that turned into eating vegan, which turned into eating nothing. It was like I wanted desperately to control something completely out of my hands and something I wanted to be untrue. I was 26 when I got my hysterectomy, not in a relationship and the finality of it was much more harder to accept than I thought it would be. It's been two years and I still have difficulty accepting it.
>
> I found out I was infertile at such a young age I never really realistically thought about it. I always dreamed I would have children and be a mother, to me it was a "when" not an "if" I became a mother. Because the hysterectomy was planned I had the option to freeze my eggs. I did think about it, but I thought the pain of watching someone else carry my baby, do something I could not, would be too far.

Breanna coped through attending counseling focusing on grief and eating disorder recovery. She journaled and joined an online community for women who have had hysterectomies. She brought up her relationship with God, and how being raised Catholic, she had always had a strong faith. She shared,

> after the hysterectomy, my faith changed and my anger with God was so profound. I go through periods where I am so mad I cannot attend church and periods where I attend extra services during the week. Emotions shift on a daily basis; some days are hard and the thought of eating feels nearly impossible. Some days are more positive.

Her thought on coping with painful emotions really struck me: "Walk into the fire," she said, "sometimes the only way to put out a fire is by letting it burn."

When she described her approach to painful emotions and her loss of hope to be a mother one day to me, a vivid image entered my head: of Breanna standing in the middle of a ring of fire and watching it as it slowly burned down and eventually extinguished. She did not stand in the fire, but did have to step over it to get to the middle space where she would not be harmed any longer by its intense heat. When the fire fully extinguished itself, I could see the ashes and the mark that the fire left on the canvas of this visual. Those scars would always be there as a representation of the pain that she endured, contacted, and lived through—the pain that she became stronger than.

Breanna's experience with infertility helps highlight that sometimes instead of trying to find water to put on the fire to extinguish it (i.e., attempting to change or decrease the emotion), we might be more inclined to sit with the feeling and let it run its course. This is akin to the acceptance and commitment therapy (ACT) technique of "riding the wave," where we follow the emotion as it comes into shore, much like a wave, and find that we won't sink and drown if we do so. I find this to be one of the most liberating and effective tools for working with difficult emotions and experiences such as shame and grief.

Clinical Tool: Working With Shame and Infertility

Research shows that working with shame and healing requires contact with the feeling of shame itself. The feeling of shame is universal and is so intense and uncomfortable that humans will naturally want to avoid it, but this takes away the opportunity for growing, learning, and healing. Effective healing comes through contacting the feeling of shame and using compassionate and acceptance based therapeutic tools to help the client navigate through this painful experience.

This tool is intended for early shame-resilience work. It is intended to explore how to show up with resilience in the face of shame as is depicted in shame resilience theory (SRT). SRT is a theory developed by Dr. Brené Brown and is "an attempt to define shame, its consequences and the ways that people (specifically women) respond to shame". According to Brené Brown, shame causes people to feel "trapped, powerless, and isolated."[12] Brown also suggests that while shame triggers can vary between individuals and cultures, there are certain triggers that are more common than others, such as "appearance and body image, sexuality, family, motherhood, parenting, professional identity and work, mental and physical health, aging, religion, speaking out, and surviving trauma."

It is shown that reinvigorating experiences where belonging, connection, and feelings of worth were present can directly reduce the power of shame. Matos and colleagues found that "shame/criticism and warmth/responsivity are not two ends of one continuum, but rather are two separate continua and clients' histories can be high or low on one or both of these." Going through the client's story and highlighting experiences of warmth, safety, comfort, belonging, and security can aid in building internal resources for the client and can help foster greater self-compassion and acceptance.[13]

Clinical Tool: Self-Compassion and Warmth Timeline

Most clients who are feeling overwhelmed by shame and criticism will focus on their story from a place of pain. They will highlight struggles, losses, shame-based experiences, and so forth. The therapist can help the client rewrite this by drawing a timeline with them. The therapist draws a line from birth to the current day. Together with the client, they slowly and carefully dictate the client's life story from a lens of strength. Where did they feel loved? What life events/situations helped foster these experiences for them? Who else was there? Create this timeline up to the present day and help the client narrate this for themselves. If they have a hard time with this or come up against a struggle, help them come up with ideas for a self-compassionate way to talk to themselves at that younger age. For example: the client experienced bullying in middle school due to the size and shape of her body. The client is very self-critical of herself during this period of her life. The client has a difficult time moving past this in the timeline. Encourage the client to talk with that younger part of herself from an "older" perspective now. How can she compassionately relate to that person's struggle and needs?[14]

Another tool, similar to the one above, is a part of Brown's shame resilience theory and helps the clients focus on "empathy, connection, power, and freedom," which are the antidotes to shame. She says there are four steps to helping clients uncover their shame and help to transform it:

1. Recognizing the personal vulnerability that led to the feelings of shame
2. Recognizing the external factors that led to the feelings of shame
3. Connecting with others to receive and offer empathy
4. Discussing and deconstructing the feelings of shame themselves.[15]

Pregorexia and the Effect of the Media

When preparing to become a mom, whether for the first time or the third, a woman naturally looks for support and belonging. What she typically finds in the media is a plethora of tabloids that discuss celebrities' pregnant and postpartum bodies and how quickly they lose the "baby weight." In her book *Does This Pregnancy Make Me Look Fat?* Claire Mysko describes our culture's obsession with celebrities' pregnancies and the countdown to when they get back to their "pre-baby body." In her research, Mysko "absolutely found that the media has an impact on a woman's obsession with her weight," and it doesn't necessarily mean she will develop an eating disorder or relapse in her recovery, but it can lead to increased anxiety around food, body, and weight during pregnancy and postpartum.[16]

Pregorexia is a term coined by the media that describes a pregnant woman's intense fear of weight gain during pregnancy, which can have a serious negative effect on the health of the fetus and newborn. She may limit her nutrition intake to the bare minimum or use compensatory behaviors that put her health at risk. It is not a clinical diagnosis and is not included in the DSM-5, and may be more common that we would expect. A woman who has anorexia, orthorexia, exercise addiction, or another an eating disorder prior to getting pregnant is at high risk of the disorder continuing into pregnancy, causing her to limit food intake, excessively exercise, and binge and purge to control her weight. This can bring up intense feelings of shame and guilt for the pregnant woman, who may be at battle with her eating disorder and herself, trying to decide which has more power and influence.

Women should normally be expected to gain between 25 and 35 pounds during pregnancy, although some gain more. While we do not have solid data about the number of pregnant women who experience pregorexia, it is estimated that 30% of pregnant women do not gain enough weight during their pregnancy, according to Dr. Ovidio Bermudez, chief medical officer at the Eating Recovery Center in Denver, Colorado. Factors such as a previous or current eating disorder or anxiety disorder in addition to pressures from the media to avoid "too much" weight gain during pregnancy can increase the risk of pregorexia. "I think you've got to be careful not to overdraw conclusions," Bermudez said. He wanted to make clear that not every woman who "struggles with weight gain" during pregnancy has an eating disorder. He continues:

> But I think there is a significant number for whom this is really another struggle, another manifestation of their eating disorder-related pathology. And those are probably the folks that are going to take it more to an extreme and the folks more likely to suffer their own health consequences as well as putting their pregnancy and the fetus, the baby, at risk.[17]

Up to two-thirds of pregnant moms do not disclose to their OB-GYN if they have a current eating disorder, and even having had a past eating disorder is not often disclosed unless asked. Society sends pregnant moms mixed messages such as you need to be "eating for two" when pregnant but "don't gain too much weight." What? How is a woman supposed to know what to do, especially if they are vulnerable to perfectionistic tendencies?

When I was pregnant, I loved my changing and growing body and found relief from any inner critic about what my body "should" be looking like. Comments from people around me, though, caused me to reflect on the strange and somewhat twisted perception that everyone else can have on a pregnant woman's body.

I got comments from my neighbor ("Are you even pregnant?") and my doctor ("I want you to eat more ice cream and fat and store some of that on your body"). (I was by no means underweight; I had never had a doctor tell me these things and they contradicted what I had told myself for so many years.) I had perfect strangers come up to me and touch my belly without asking permission. How is this okay, when it's not okay at all when one is not pregnant? When you are pregnant, your belly is out there for all comments, judgments, or opinions—vulnerability that one cannot change or hide.

For a woman who has an eating disorder, this exposure of her body combined with her body changing in ways she cannot control can trigger maladaptive coping mechanisms and behaviors such as restriction or purging (through laxatives, exercise, or throwing up).

Emily, now 33, gained 32 pounds during her first pregnancy, and her doctor said she "was right on track." Emily had struggled with anorexia and exercise bulimia as a teenager when she was a track star and became hyper-focused on weight as a means to achieving faster running scores. She had been to therapy for this issue and felt "recovered" when she was 23.

She delivered a healthy baby but soon began restricting her food intake and exercising above her doctor's suggestions. When a few years later she became pregnant again, she told herself "she was not going to let THAT happen again," meaning gaining "that much weight" and "being that out of control." This disordered mindset was fed by her perceived feeling of being out of control during pregnancy and coupled with the stress of caring for a newborn and a toddler, this coping strategy felt "comforting." She did not disclose this plan to her doctor and began having some bleeding when she was about 11 weeks pregnant. Her doctors feared a miscarriage and told her to rest and make sure she was getting lots of fluids and nutrition. Emily continued to exercise excessively and cut her calories to a "non-pregnant" number, and when she was 25 weeks pregnant her baby was measuring small. She felt so much shame and fear. She loved her baby so much and did not want to hurt her, but also felt very out of control with her exercise obsession and "could not stop." The shame and guilt about her behaviors kept her from disclosing to her doctor just how much she was actually exercising and the vicious cycle was reinforced.

Shame slinks under the hood of the car; it escapes detection externally and is fiercely protected and hidden on the inside. She thought: "what mom would do this to her unborn baby?" In Emily's case, the cycle was as shown in Figure 5.1:

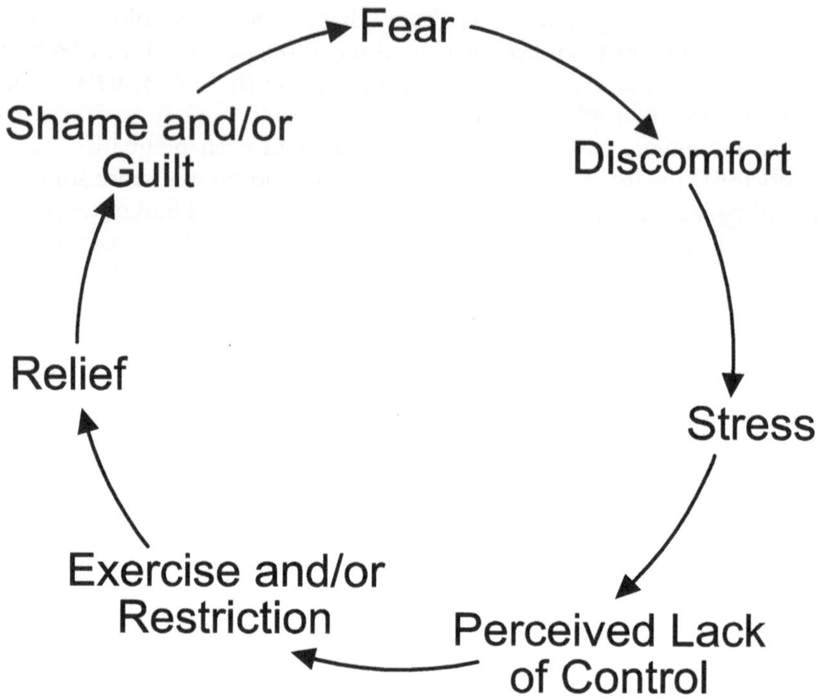

Figure 5.1 An example of the fear-shame cycle that can trigger disordered coping mechanisms

Tip for therapists: Look out for warning signs. If you are treating a pregnant woman who has a history of an eating disorder, check in with her about her attitudes toward her pregnancy, her body and herself. Normal conversations she would be having with herself and her loved ones would involve what to name the baby, how to decorate the nursery, and what to pack in her hospital bag; these should mostly be focus on her baby, not herself. While some worry and anxiety is certainly normal for any expectant or new mom, if the pregnant mom is consumed with worry and obsession about herself, such as "how am I going to lose the weight?" "when can I start exercising again after birth? (in an obsessive manner, not a healthy curiosity) and "am I going to still be loveable after I go through all of this?" these might be signs that she is at risk for a postpartum mood disorder or eating disorder.

Emily gained only 18 pounds in her second pregnancy and delivered her son prematurely and at a low birth weight. They struggled to develop a nursing relationship and her son began having seizures when he was only 6 weeks old. The doctors feel that this might have been due to the poor nutrition that he received when he was in utero.

Emily blamed herself for her son's health problems: "I feel like I did this to him." She struggled to bond with her son because every time she looked at him or held him she was reminded of the behaviors and shame that caused her to treat her body the way she did during pregnancy. She returned to eating disorder treatment and has now fully recovered. Her son is now healthy and thriving and they have a very close relationship. But so many other new moms live with this shame every day, wondering if they could have done something different to prevent their child from having pain and suffering, or beating themselves up for choices they made in the past.

Other moms can report a different experience, equally painful. Entering pregnancy at a higher weight than they felt comfortable with, the increased weight gain during pregnancy can lead to feelings of shame and criticism. Britney, age 39, was in recovery from binge eating disorder and told by her doctors to gain only 5–10 pounds because "she was so heavy" when she got pregnant. For a woman who is at a higher BMI when she gets pregnant, the amount of recommended weight gain can vary depending on several different factors. Most doctors will recommend she gain a minimal amount of weight (5–15 pounds), but these doctors might also miss the shaming message this can send to their patients. If a doctor can adopt a Health at Every Size approach,[18] they can treat their patient with respect and see them from a holistic perspective, and not just a weight perspective. For women who have a history of an eating disorder, this topic and approach is especially vulnerable.

Britney experienced confusion and feelings of helplessness and struggled to follow her body's cues out of fear of gaining "too much weight" and disappointing her medical team. She also desperately did not want to harm her growing baby. She delivered a healthy baby girl but felt shame about her weight gain (which was more than 10 pounds), and she struggled to lose weight after giving birth due to the demands of being a new mother and the shame she felt about her body.

Britney's doctors focused almost exclusively on her weight and did not talk with her about her health as a whole person. They did not ask about stress levels and how she was doing at managing them. While in a "normal pregnancy" a woman "usually gains up to 20 pounds," this is different for each woman and each pregnancy. Every body is different, yet our society's medical evaluation system (and BMI) does not leave room for this. Britney felt shame at already being at a higher weight. Because of the power imbalance in the doctor-patient relationship, Britney felt pressured to "please her doctor," even if that meant straying from her body's natural cues.

Britney became pregnant again 2 years later and vowed to "do it differently this time." She "controlled" her weight during pregnancy and received accolades from her doctors who told her "she might leave the hospital with a flat tummy because she did a good job managing her weight during pregnancy." This positive encouragement was addictive. She came to her 6-week postpartum checkup 32 pounds lighter than her pre-pregnancy weight. She felt great about this, but also shame at the measures that she had to take to achieve this, which involved severe restriction of her food intake, which can put her body at risk of being unable to produce adequate breast milk if she is nursing. A postpartum body needs time and patience to change after the intensely demanding job of growing a baby inside of it and then birthing the baby. Severe weight loss postpartum affects the body's muscle strength and can put a woman at long-term risk for health problems down the road. Britney ultimately explored all of this with her therapist and felt anger at her doctors for encouraging such unhealthy behavior and for not understanding her situation.

Women are taught by society and the patriarchy to put themselves down. We always need to be smaller, quieter, and more docile. This undercurrent of repression can reveal itself during pregnancy as well, where a woman desires to stay small or to please their doctor who holds so much power. "Instead of celebrating weight loss," says Jennifer Gaudiani, a prominent Denver physician who specializes in eating disorders, "how about we celebrate the things we cannot post a selfie about?"

When Shame Seeps in to Your Relationship

Attachment wounds can cut deep in a relationship: loss, infidelity, trauma, mental health issues, infertility, addiction. These are a few of the conditions that can become a third party in a couple's attachment and secure connection with each other. As we explore the experience of infertility, pregnancy, and eating disorders we must touch on the way the experience of shame can strain the safety, security, and closeness of a couple.

In our first population, we have found that the inability to conceive a child can induce stress in an individual as well as a couple. A 2004 study by Chen et al. of the psychological effects of infertility reported that for women receiving medical treatment for infertility, "40.2% have a psychiatric disorder with generalized anxiety disorder being the most prevalent (23.2%) followed by major depression (17.0%) and dysthymia disorder (9.8%)."[19] It was found that more than half of the couples studied were able to cope effectively with the infertility experience, but others struggled to cope individually and as a couple with the emotional distress of the experience, thus underlying the need for psychological interventions.

The condition of infertility elicits complex psychological responses. Here we find that learned gender roles can sometimes come into play and influence how one internalizes the experience.

Many women have heard a message since childhood and adolescence about the "important role of being a mother," and they find that when they grow up and get married, they feel the urge to begin having their own family. For women, this is often a central component to their identity in their childbearing years, influenced by biological factors, family of origin values, and their own personal values and societal expectation. When their desire to have a child does not produce the result they were hoping for, a sense of loss of identity and feelings of defectiveness and incompetence are quite often experienced.[20]

Toni, 36, who with her husband have gone through three cycles of IVF in an attempt to get pregnant, shares:

> What's really frustrating is when women of all ages (especially older women) ask me: why don't you have children? Don't you want to have a child? When they know nothing about my situation. There are so many things wrong with this. First off, what if I don't choose to have children? Does that make me less of a woman? Less important to society? And secondly, which is actually my experience, what if I have been trying to get pregnant and am struggling to conceive? Why is it anyone's business other than my husband and my own what our fertility choices are? It's like when you are a woman of a childbearing age your fertility status becomes fair game for everyone to know about, assume things about, and ask/judge about. It's unnerving.

Eating disorders can contribute to feelings similar to this internalization of "brokenness," and if both an ED and infertility exist concurrently, the experience of shame becomes more likely. Shame has been referred to as an important emotion in the experience of infertility, related to a sense of loss of control over the body, feelings of personal exposure, of being a sexual failure or defective in some way.[21] Couples trying to cope with shame, infertility, an eating disorder, and other psychological pain can experience disconnect in their relationship as they try to navigate through it.

I spoke with Anna, a 34-year-old professional who has been married to Eric for 5 years. She grew up with two older sisters, both of whom have young families of their own now, and describes herself "as the most motherly and nurturing of her siblings." She has always been very career-focused and had entered residential treatment for anorexia binge-purge type when she was 20. She states that treatment was successful and "she had a few slip ups over the years, one of them lasting a few months, but that she has been relatively stable" since she got married to Eric in 2013. Anna describes her commitment to her recovery as "closely aligned with her desire to have a family with Eric." She also calls herself "a recovering perfectionist" and says that her internal world is "hectic and chaotic sometimes" and that she "is pretty hard on herself about many things." She attends therapy and finds that focusing on increasing her self-compassion is effective in navigating around the critical mind.

With her job in real estate successful and solid, Anna and Eric decided they wanted to try to have a family in 2015. Anna had been taking prenatal vitamins, following a healthy diet, and striving for a normal and relaxed relationship with exercise (which at one point had been an ED behavior). She stopped taking birth control, but after 3 months she did not have a regular period. Doctors ran tests but could find nothing that could prevent her from being fertile and getting pregnant. They also said "they didn't really know and need to continue to run tests and try different medications." The not knowing and nonlinear track that this process began to feed Anna's anxiety and stress. Month after month, Anna felt her hope and excitement slowly decrease. She began pulling away from Eric and distanced herself as her negative, critical mind was in overdrive. Shame that she had felt within her eating disorder years began to seep back in.

Shame is tied very closely to one's identity and is associated with the internal experience of the self as undesirable, defective, worthless, and powerless.[22] It has been divided into two types of shame: internal and external. Gilbert describes it as "fundamentally an experience of the self linked to how one believes one exists in the mind of the others."

Shame types can be delineated based on thoughts, behaviors, and attention focus. External shame is focused on the external environment that one dwells in, in which they believe they exist negatively in the minds of others, that they are flawed, inadequate, or inferior. Internal shame relates to one's own private internal world. They may judge themselves for these same things and experience these same feelings of inadequacy and being flawed. External and internal shame have been found in some cases to be linked and in others to be independent constructs.[23]

What we find here is the connection between internalized shame (self-devaluation and self-criticism) and how it relates to both the experience of infertility and of past and current eating disorder behaviors. Anna sank deep into the depths of shame and despair, linking her eating disorder past to her current experience of infertility and "feeling out of control." She experienced the reemergence of her harsh critic voice that had dominated much of her conscious life during the time of her eating disorder.

This critical mind drew a connection between her past eating disorder and the self-destructive behaviors that it caused her to have, such as starving herself and then throwing up the small amounts of food she did eat (which felt like "binges" to her at the time), in addition to intense exercising and her current diagnosis of infertility. Her negative and self-devaluing mind screamed at her that "it's all your fault that you can't have a baby. You did this to yourself. You don't deserve to be a parent." Without anyone else hearing this and little opportunity to challenge this strong force of a mind, Anna withdrew into a world of self-devaluation and hatred.

She began to isolate herself from Eric, her family, and her friends—all of whom she had in the past confided in about her struggles and triumphs. She also began to feel angry at people who appeared to have what Anna so desperately wanted. Pregnant women would trigger Anna to feel anger at herself and at them, and she began to avoid places where she might see a pregnant person (which was everywhere). She then felt shame and embarrassment for these feelings and reactions.

Anna falls in the category of someone experiencing "shame proneness." Tangney and colleagues have distinguished between "state shame," which refers to shame feelings that someone feels in a certain situation, such as being dishonest with your spouse about how much money you spent on a shopping trip; and "shame proneness," which is defined as an innate disposition to experience shame and may arise for early childhood experiences.[24] Anna's current experience of feeling out of control and unable to grasp something that she values so much triggered past feelings from her childhood and adolescence in which she felt inadequate, unworthy, and a failure. Anna's mother was highly critical of her and pushed her to "be her best," which Anna internalized as not being good enough if she could not attain a perfect score, grade, or body type. This developed into self-focused perfectionism, which tainted her every move and choice as she grew up. She wanted to be "good enough," to be loved as the narrative of her childhood had reinforced to her, and this meant being "the best" at any cost.

Feelings of not being good enough for her mother or to be accepted at school seeped into feelings of shame and contributed to her food restriction in high school to "be thin and fit in," as her mind told her. As adult Anna in her current situation had the awareness that going back into her ED would not help and would in reality take her further away from her goal of being a mother, she felt helpless as to what to do next. Her shame intensified as she continued to grasp at straws to attempt to figure out next steps. Eric was also experiencing his own grief and loss at the infertility diagnosis and in addition felt as if he was losing his wife, too. He felt despair at Anna's pain and suffering and also helplessness at how to connect with the woman he loved unconditionally and who he felt was slipping away from him.

Research on shame and shame proneness has highlighted the link between the onset of depression and/or anxiety and these intense internal experiences. Kristin Neff, a prominent researcher on self-compassion, describes self-judgment as "being harshly self-critical in instances of failure or pain, perceiving one's experiences as separate from the larger human experience and over-identifying with painful thoughts and feelings."[25] She continues to explain that when dealing with suffering or feelings of inadequacy or failure, self-judgmental individuals tend to belittle their own pain or berate themselves with self-criticism. This in turn may initiate coping strategies such as disordered eating, substance abuse, or other avoidant numbing strategies.

Clinical Tool: Allowing the Pain

Many times when we experience pain and suffering, we spend so much energy trying to identify the "why" and to write the story of the causes of our pain. This is one way that our minds attempt to help us—by thinking so hard about the reason for the pain and in many instances finding a person or situation to attach the pain to. We then might get some temporary relief from the actual feeling of the pain. In many cases, the pain feels unbearable, and there is a time and a use for distraction. Some ideas for mindful distraction are coloring, sewing, writing, making art, playing a game, going for a walk, and listening to music.

However, without interrupting the distraction and contacting the feeling (pain) underneath, we put ourselves at risk for further suffering and the development of maladaptive coping strategies to "numb" the pain. In acceptance and commitment therapy (ACT), this is called experiential avoidance, and it can go out of control and create a whole new problem such as substance abuse, eating disorders, depression, anxiety, and much more.

Anna worked with her therapist on trying to allow and feel her pain instead of explain it or cognitively detach from it. This technique needs to be done in a safe place (i.e., in the context of a safe therapeutic relationship) and with the client being in charge of intensity and timing. The goal of the tool is to allow the somatic experience in Anna's body of whatever she feels and making room for self-compassion, self-kindness, and self-acceptance to appear in the place of shame and self-judgment. Or if it is difficult to replace the negative internal experiences, she can try to use expansion and "make room" around them for an additional experience such as self-kindness or curiosity. Expansion can also mean allowing or accepting an experience instead of rejecting it. It might be aligned with flexibility and leaning-in instead of rigidity and closing down.

Anna writes on a large piece of paper all of the thoughts and "stories" that she has about her pain: "it's because of my ED; I shouldn't feel this way; (subjective perceptions/judgments); I deserve to feel this way, I'm a horrible person; I'm a failure." These occur when one becomes fused with their thoughts and feelings and there is little room to challenge them or look at them a different way.

Also facts: "I have had three rounds of IVF and they were unsuccessful; I struggled with an ED for 12 years; I am in a loving and compassionate marriage" (facts/objective). Writing these out and whatever comes to mind in a "bubble cloud." The therapist tracks Anna's subjective and emotive experience as she writes these. She checks in with her. After they write these for 10 minutes or so, her therapist asks her to rate her pain on a scale of 1 to 10. Her therapist helps her to stay with the feeling and to acknowledge that it is part of her healing process but also gives Anna permission to stop and use a distraction whenever she would like. Anna is in charge and is encouraged to advocate for herself and her body's needs. Her therapist encourages her to let her body do what it needs to stay with the pain (act it out, cry, scream, make art, etc.). They then create new statements based on feeling—I feel pain, I feel angry, I feel sad, and so forth, without any judgment of the feeling.

Anna's therapist encourages her to notice what happens with the feelings in her body when she sits with them instead of avoids them. Do they change shape? Size? Intensity? Color? Texture?

When we feel our feelings, they transform. They are no longer stagnant. They are like water, always moving and flowing—sometimes in a giant wave, sometimes in a gentle ripple. The goal of this tool is not to make Anna feel better necessarily (although if that is the outcome, that is positive) but to help her see that she has power and choice in her body and with her emotions, and to hopefully see them from a new and less labeling or judgmental perspective. She then could develop a new relationship with her experience.

Anna and Eric are continuing on their fertility journey and are now trying IUI (intrauterine insemination) and are hopeful that this will result in a pregnancy. Anna reports feelings slightly less attached to the shame and has fewer "spirals into the depths," as she calls it. She is trying to move forward with a slight distance to the process and to hold hope for each stage of their journey. Anna and Eric are in couples counseling to work on reconnecting in their new reality. Anna feels that Eric "doesn't understand what she's feeling," but she is trying to open up to him and let him in. She accesses parts of her past ED recovery as she reaches out and attempts to connect with Eric, even when she feels shame, grief, and sadness. Her resiliency builds and their bond becomes deeper and more complex.

Perfectionism and anxiety can set the stage for shame and guilt to seep in if life does not go "according to plan," which may be a significant trigger for women who have perfectionistic qualities. The concept of "radical acceptance" can play a part in offering a new perspective to adjusting to life situations that are not ideal, and even in the imperfection a new sense of peace can be found. This chapter has explored the role of vulnerability in helping to build resiliency for individuals and for couples who are enduring fertility challenges and/or eating disorders. When self-compassion and openness with oneself and one's partner are present, a path toward acceptance and healing is possible.

Considerations for Therapists

1. Differentiating between "state shame" and "shame proneness" can be significant when treating clients who are susceptible to internalizing situations in a negative capacity. What traits, behaviors, or

patterns would you look for in clients to define what they are experiencing, and how would you approach this in the treatment realm?
2. To do this work we need to "walk the talk." When have you felt feelings of shame? How did you recognize this and cope with it?
3. What are additional tools or interventions that can be used to help a pregnant woman who is struggling to take care of herself and her body amid the "thin ideal"?

Notes

1. Brown, B. (2015). *Daring greatly: How the courage to be vulnerable transforms the way we live, love, parent, and lead*. London: Penguin Life.
2. Perfectionism (psychology). (2018, December 24). Retrieved from https://en.wikipedia.org/wiki/Perfectionism_(psychology)
3. Benson, E. (2003, November). *The many faces of perfectionism*. Retrieved from www.apa.org/monitor/nov03/manyfaces.aspx
4. Benson, E. (2003, November). *The many faces of perfectionism*. Retrieved from www.apa.org/monitor/nov03/manyfaces.aspx
5. Ruggeri, A. (2018, February 21). *Future: The dangerous downsides of perfectionism*. Retrieved from www.bbc.com/future/story/20180219-toxic-perfectionism-is-on-the-rise
6. Statistics & Research on Eating Disorders. (2018, September 14). Retrieved December 28, 2018, from www.nationaleatingdisorders.org/statistics-research-eating-disorders
7. Ruggeri, A. (2018, February 21). Future: The dangerous downsides of perfectionism. Retrieved from www.bbc.com/future/story/20180219-toxic-perfectionism-is-on-the-rise
8. Benson, E. (2003, November). *The many faces of perfectionism*. Retrieved from www.apa.org/monitor/nov03/manyfaces.aspx
9. Andreyeva, T., Puhl, R. M., & Brownell, K. D. (2008). changes in perceived weight discrimination among Americans, 1995–1996 through 2004–2006. *Obesity*, *16*, 1129–1134. https://doi.org/10.1038/oby.2008.35
10. Golden, N. H., Schneider, M., & Wood, C. (2016). preventing obesity and eating disorders in adolescents. *Pediatrics*, *138*(3). https://doi.org/10.1542/peds.2016-1649
11. Brach, T. (2012). *Radical acceptance: Awakening the love that heals fear and shame*. London: Ebury Digital.
12. Home. (2018). Retrieved December 30, 2018, from www.brenebrown.com/
13. Matos, M., Gouveia, J. P., & Duarte, C. (2015). Constructing a self protected against shame: The importance of warmth and safeness memories and feelings on the association between shame memories and depression. *International Journal of Psychology and Psychological Therapy*, *15*(3), 317–335.
14. Adapted from LeJeune, J. (2016). *20 science-based recommendations for therapy with highly self-critical or shame-prone clients*. Retrieved December 30, 2018, from www.actwithcompassion.com/20_science_based_recommendations_for_therapy_with_highly_self_critical_or_shame_prone_clients
15. Home. (2018). Retrieved December 30, 2018, from www.brenebrown.com/
16. Mysko, C., & Amadeï, M. (2009). *Does this pregnancy make me look fat?: The essential guide to loving your body before and after baby*. Deerfield Beach, FL: Health Communications.
17. Wallace, K. (2013, November 20). *'Pregorexia': Extreme dieting by pregnant women*. Retrieved December 30, 2018, from www.cnn.com/2013/11/20/living/pregnant-dieting-pregorexia-moms/index.html

18. Health at Every Size. (2018). Retrieved December 28, 2018, from https://haescommunity.com/
19. Galhardo, A., Pinto-Gouveia, J., Cunha, M., & Matos, M. (2011). The impact of shame and self-judgment on psychopathology in infertile patients. *Human Reproduction*, *26*(9), 2408–2414. https://doi.org/10.1093/humrep/der209
20. Galhardo, A., Pinto-Gouveia, J., Cunha, M., & Matos, M. (2011). The impact of shame and self-judgment on psychopathology in infertile patients. *Human Reproduction*, *26*(9), 2408–2414. https://doi.org/10.1093/humrep/der209
21. Galhardo, A., Pinto-Gouveia, J., Cunha, M., & Matos, M. (2011). The impact of shame and self-judgment on psychopathology in infertile patients. *Human Reproduction*, *26*(9), 2408–2414. https://doi.org/10.1093/humrep/der209
22. Galhardo, A., Pinto-Gouveia, J., Cunha, M., & Matos, M. (2011). The impact of shame and self-judgment on psychopathology in infertile patients. *Human Reproduction*, *26*(9), 2408–2414. https://doi.org/10.1093/humrep/der209
23. Galhardo, A., Pinto-Gouveia, J., Cunha, M., & Matos, M. (2011). The impact of shame and self-judgment on psychopathology in infertile patients. *Human Reproduction*, *26*(9), 2408–2414. https://doi.org/10.1093/humrep/der209
24. Galhardo, A., Pinto-Gouveia, J., Cunha, M., & Matos, M. (2011). The impact of shame and self-judgment on psychopathology in infertile patients. *Human Reproduction*, *26*(9), 2408–2414. https://doi.org/10.1093/humrep/der209
25. Neff, K. (2015). *Self-compassion: Stop beating yourself up and leave insecurity behind*. New York: William Morrow.

6 What the Medical Community Needs to Know to Support Clients

If you try to lose weight—maybe 10, 15 pounds—then you'd have a better chance of getting pregnant.

Make sure to keep an eye on your weight while you're pregnant; you don't want to gain too much. Maybe buy a scale to track this?

You're thin, there's no reason that you should have any issues getting pregnant.

You did a good job with your weight during your pregnancy; you should be able to have a flat stomach by the time of your 6-week postpartum checkup.

If you're not menstruating regularly, let's put you on birth control pills, that should help. It also could be PCOS, and if you lose weight that probably will fix it.

These are all statements that patients have heard from their doctor when they go in to discuss fertility, while they are pregnant, or have recently become a parent. Many of these statements were made with minimal assessment of emotional, social, or psychological aspects to the patient's physical presenting issue or concern. Of the women that I interviewed, more than 50% stated that their doctors focused primarily on their weight (loss/gain) as an assessment for health and omitted or brushed over questions about their overall wellness.

This can stigmatize patients who do not fit into the "ideal" picture of health, especially those in larger bodies, and lead them to avoid going to the doctor or opening up about more vulnerable topics. Several of the women in my study shared that their medical providers pushed weight loss surgery as a means to improve their fertility status (and overall health) with minimal focus on addressing other factors that may be at play such as socioeconomic status, trauma, depression/anxiety, eating disorders, and life stressors. A few women shared that they were "readily approved" for bariatric surgery when they asked their doctors about it, and a source from within the healthcare industry said, "[for the insurance companies], it's all about money."

It is important to assess emotional and psychological factors that may be impacting a woman's fertility, especially if she is in a larger body as this population is often "invisibilized" and the focus is on their weight specifically. If a woman suffers from an eating disorder such as BED, the behaviors may affect her body's ability to conceive and sustain a pregnancy. Weight loss alone will not address the deeper issues contributing to infertility.

On the television show *This Is Us*, the character of Kate, who is in a larger body, is diagnosed with polycystic ovary syndrome (PCOS) and also struggles with binge eating. She visits a fertility clinic and is told by her doctor that due to her weight she has a very slim chance of getting pregnant and that the risk of taking her on as an IVF patient is too high for the doctor to agree to. The doctor focuses strictly on her weight as the issue instead of asking her about other factors that may be present that could affect her eating behaviors, health, and fertility status.

This is a television show that depicts the real-life experience of women all over the world. Kate feels shame, channels this inward, and shuts herself off to her husband and family. Kate's relationship with her body has been a lifelong struggle, influenced by her mother's comments, tragic loss of her father, and other situations that she has turned to food to cope with. When she and her husband Toby want to start a family, she is again met with weight stigma, which seems to have followed her entire life. Because of her weight she is deemed too much of a risk for IVF; this is a missed opportunity for the show to talk about weight stigma and fat shaming and to look at the whole picture, not just Kate's weight.

When the doctor decides she will "take that chance" with Kate, the power and influence of the medical community over the patient is evident. Kate ultimately does get pregnant from IVF amid her whole family being concerned about this being "too dangerous" of a procedure due to her weight. Perhaps this doctor could have asked Kate more about health in many different aspects: how she likes to take care of herself, what her body tells her, how she practices movement, her history with mental health issues, if she is getting support for her eating disorder, and so forth. This is just a TV show and not real life, but this type of encounter mimics real-life doctor visits every day and the show reaches millions of viewers. Numerous women told me that their doctors never asked them about an eating disorder history. Many were applauded for being in a healthy weight range; many were scolded for not being in one.

In this world of weight stigma and fat-shaming, is it any wonder that only about one-third of patients disclose to their OB-GYN or fertility doctor about a past or a current eating disorder?[1] And yet, upwards of 21% of patients at fertility clinics have a current or a past eating disorder.[2]

What are the reasons for this? What is influencing these patients and preventing them from being more open?

I had the opportunity to interview Denver's prominent internist who specializes in eating disorders, Jennifer Gaudiani, MD, CEDS, FAED. She is the founder and medical director of the Gaudiani Clinic, a unique outpatient medical clinic specifically dedicated to adolescents and adults of all shapes and sizes who have eating disorders or a history of an eating disorder. Dr. Gaudiani also recently published a book, *Sick Enough: A Guide to the Medical Complications of Eating Disorders* (Routledge, 2018), which offers patients, their families, and clinicians a comprehensive, accessible review of the medical issues that arise from eating disorders.

Her clinic is founded on a Health at Every Size (HAES) perspective,[3] which means that it celebrates body diversity and honors health at any size that a body feels best in. She offered me her perspective on the barriers to care that patients encounter when they have an eating disorder and are seeking to get pregnant or are currently pregnant.

Literature review provided a foundation for women's attitudes toward broaching the subject of having an eating disorder with their medical team. Bye et al. performed the first comprehensive study to "specifically explore the perspectives of women and health professionals on the barriers to identifying eating disorders during and after pregnancy."[4] The main findings of their study were that women were hesitant to disclose a current or past eating disorder due to risk of encountering stigma about the disorder. Health professionals expressed a similar hesitancy to ask and explore this topic with patients due to lack of confidence and training in the area of eating disorders.

Stigma is found to be one of the most common and prominent factors that impacts women from seeking out mental health care. Stigma involves "perceived and experienced stereotyping, prejudice, and discrimination to the detriment of the targeted group."[5] Weight stigma is a prominent influence in today's society and is reinforced by antiobesity campaigns, which result in further ostracizing and shaming of people who are in larger bodies.

There is a helpful way to distinguish between guilt, which is more externalized and shame, which is more internalized. Guilt says, "I feel badly about something I have done." Shame says, "I am bad. I am wrong." Guilt can be rectified and forgiven; shame seeps deep into the "swampland of the soul," according to Brené Brown, and sticks to our very core. It is toxic.

Attitudes that are influenced by stigma (such as fat is bad, fat people are lazy and stupid, etc.) can lead to feelings of guilt and shame in the targeted populations and can cause an individual to feel a sense of personal responsibility for their actions, even if their eating disorder behaviors are not in their control. Shame seeps deeper, and they may feel that there is something fundamentally wrong with them as a person. This experience can lead to patients not wanting to disclose their eating disorder to their doctor, as eating disorders thrive on shame.

Short Facts:

- Patients with eating disorders seek treatment at fertility clinics at almost twice the rate of patients without Eds.[6]
- Patients with eating disorders get pregnant unintentionally at twice the rate as those who do not have EDs.[7] "Eggs happen," says Dr. Gaudiani. This is in part due to lack of medical awareness about sex and fertility, which should be given by doctors.
- One-fourth of women with bulimia who are pregnant end their pregnancy in abortion, which is higher than the general population.[8]
- In women who have BED, almost 50% of their pregnancies end in miscarriage.
- Women with BED are at risk of having higher birth weight babies because of insulin being a growth hormone. This can lead to birth complications and some potential health issues for baby and mom.
- Women with AN risk growth retardation, premature delivery, and other risks to their baby due to malnourishment (not genetic).
- When a woman's body is severely malnourished, no matter her body shape or size, her brain assesses and determines that a famine is going on. It goes into self-preservation mode (we can call this "caveman brain") where her primal instincts will do anything possible to prevent death. Her ovaries will shrink to prepuberty size, hormone production will slow or halt, and her brain will tell her body "it's not safe to have a baby right now. We don't have enough resources available to survive."
- In males with an eating disorder, their brain will reduce or halt testosterone production to preadolescent levels for the same reasons.
- There is a higher chance for pregnancy complications such as miscarriage or fetus deformity (not genetically based) if a woman's body is malnourished during pregnancy.
- An ED can go into "remission" during pregnancy, however at 18 months postpartum there is a 40%–70% relapse rate in this population.[9]
- A flood of "happy hormones" can trigger feeling of being "fine" and not needing therapy or support anymore during pregnancy, which can put the mother and baby at risk for relapse and struggle postpartum.
- In a Swedish study, 20.7% of patients at a fertility clinic had a current or past eating disorder, and none disclosed this fact to their doctor.[10]

Why? I think it points back to weight and eating disorder (and all mental illness) stigma and fearing judgment or inappropriate response from their provider. Also, many patients have an allegiance to their eating disorder and have a deep fear or ambivalence of letting it go.

The best and safest thing to do for a woman desiring to have a baby is to wait until she is physically and emotionally well before proceeding to try to conceive.

For patients who are terrified of gaining weight in order for their bodies to reach a healthy state, the idea of getting fertility treatments can seem promising, as they can take fertility drugs and not have to do the deep recovery work. And their doctor may buy into the thin ideal.

Barriers to Identifying Eating Disorders in the Medical Setting

> I'm continually astounded by the damaging power of physician internalized size stigma.
>
> —Jennifer Gaudiani, MD

In the Bye et al. study, the most prominent one of its kind, five barriers to identifying an eating disorder in the pregnancy or postnatal period *as perceived by patients* were identified. They were:

1. *Stigma*: Some women described feeling judged by health professionals based on their physical appearance, as illustrated by one woman who stated:

   I was overweight according to my BMI. I didn't think they would believe me to tell them I had an actual problem. I was patronized by more than one healthcare professional who tried to educate me on nutrition. I got the impression they thought I was just lazy and ate junk food all of the time when this wasn't the case. I felt they were too judgmental to approach.

2. *Lack of opportunity*: Women described feeling there was not time or an opportunity to disclose this information to their doctor, nor that they had developed enough of a rapport with them to be able to open up: "they didn't ask and it wasn't raised as a concern." Just as with other topics that are uncomfortable and painful, eating disorders can dwell in a "don't ask, don't tell" atmosphere which stays shrouded in secrecy and shame. Of the women whose medical team did assess for eating disorders, they reported "poor follow up and follow through" in subsequent appointments, leaving the women to feel isolated in their experience.

   On the flip side, Bye's study found that many medical professionals felt they did not have enough training or knowledge to comprehensively address or treat the issue. Hence the lack of confidence for many in how to follow up or assess further for disordered eating during the fertility treatment process.

3. *Preference for self-management*: Some women reported not sharing info about their ED because they preferred to "manage it on their own." They might have had the issue for so long that it felt like a part of them or they did not believe that anyone else could effectively help them with it. This is also closely aligned with denial of the severity or impact of the eating disorder on their functioning. "I don't like to talk about it and think I can manage on my own," and "I just wanted to deal with it myself." The eating disorder identity becomes triggered when a new identity arises, and may appear larger and stronger, reminding the woman of why she "needs" it and does not need to let it go during her pregnancy: "I don't really like to talk about it. I have had some sort of disordered eating for a very long time it is very much part of me and no one else's business."
4. *Current ED symptomatology*: Some women felt as if they did not need to disclose because "they have been fine for a while" or feel that their ED is "not a problem [anymore]." With the high rate of remission of ED symptoms during pregnancy, some patients may feel that their ED is not an issue or warranting of bringing up to their medical team. This may increase the risk of the team not detecting or assessing for medical complications of the eating disorder as well as the patient feeling that she is "well" and ending her therapeutic support right when she needs it the most.
5. *Illness awareness*: Many women did not recognize their symptoms as that of an eating disorder or did not think it was a problem. Interestingly, this was particularly prevalent in women with binge eating disorder as some had categorized their binge eating behaviors as general overeating. One patient said: "Binge eating doesn't seem like that big of an issue and I've never seen it as an eating disorder before," pointing to the need for more education about eating disorders and the normalization of disordered eating behaviors in our society, whether it is restriction or binge eating. Another woman shared: "I have only really just recognised that I have an issue and at the time I was pregnant did not realise. I just thought I was a greedy person."[11]

Health professionals were also interviewed to discuss from *their perspective* the barriers perceived to providing adequate care to fertility patients with an eating disorder history. Four main themes emerged here:

1. *System constraints*: In Bye's study of health professionals, all of those interviewed reported minimal or absent focus or training on EDs during their clinical education with one participant noting, "I know what an eating disorder is but I've not come across it through my health visitor training." Much of the knowledge of eating disorders had to be pieced together from training on other taught topics, as one midwife shared: "it would be linked to other mental health or BMI."

This is problematic due to the deep-rooted weight bias that plagues the medical community, and BMI is a measurement focusing purely on numbers and not including any other health factors. Learning about eating disorders from the BMI (weight and numbers) perspective instead of a holistic assessment of mental, emotional, physical, and systemic factors can prove to be damaging to the treatment of a woman in a fertility clinic who has an eating disorder. Of health professionals who did get some eating disorder education, they felt it was an introduction and didn't give them tools for how to approach EDs during and after pregnancy. One midwife said: "I don't know whether it was actually mentioned apart from refer to a dietician, there wasn't really any practical advice of what we need to do."

2. *Recognition of role*: Health professionals interviewed here cited a strong desire to inquire about eating disorders when meeting with patients, but noted that due to their lack of confidence and limited competence on diagnosing and treating mental health disorders they determined their role to be more "advisory and supportive" than intervening. They felt that their role should be focused primarily on the physical well-being of the mother and fetus and not the mother's mental health. This is a missed opportunity for further assessment and intervention of treating any mental disorder or mental health issue that may be interfering with the mother's quality of life, which then can affect the physical and mental well-being of her child. "We would be just making sure that the baby was growing adequately . . . and then leaving the woman well alone in a way just focusing on the wellbeing of the baby."
3. *Personal attitudes*: The personal experiences, beliefs, attitudes, and values of the health professional will influence how she assesses for eating disorders and other mental health issues in her patients. One midwife interviewed shared that she would feel more uncomfortable to inquire about an eating disorder in women who were overweight than in women who were underweight. I wonder if this is due to weight stigma and discomfort discussing weight and eating disorders, and also if this speaks to the invisibility and mis-assessment of eating disorders in normal to overweight women.
4. *Stigma and taboo*: Eating disorders are not desirable topics for anyone to bring up. There is much stigma associated with them, just as with domestic violence or suicidality and health professionals expressed hesitancy to assess them. For many women who are pregnant, they may have a fear (both rational and irrational) that if they discussed their mental health issues with their doctor this equals their baby being taken away by social services. Both the patient and the doctor may skirt the topic: "You've never had any eating disorders, have you? Great. Moving right along."[12]

In reviewing these barriers to treatment of pregnant and postpartum women who have an eating disorder, it is little surprise that so many EDs go undiagnosed during the process of getting and being pregnant. Many of these women are in an invisibilized population; they may be at a "healthy weight" and therefore not perceived to be unwell, or they may have atypical anorexia, bulimia, or binge eating disorder that doesn't fit strictly into the DSM categories.

Dr. Gaudiani described a common type of patient seen in fertility clinics: this woman and her partner can go to multiple fertility clinics and for 2 years go through a very expensive and heartbreaking process of trying to become pregnant. This patient does not recall being stopped by her doctor(s) and told:

> I will not treat you. You need to stop exercising, improve eating and nutrition, gain [xx pounds] and try naturally during that time period. It's not safe for me to give you fertility treatment because your body cannot sustain a pregnancy right now.

Doctors have so much power, and oftentimes they do not intervene when they could help. In this case it is unsafe to treat patients due to disordered eating and exercising behaviors that need to be assessed by the patient's medical team. This is different from the example of Kate in *This Is Us*, where her weight was pinpointed as the reason for withholding treatment.

A lack of intervention or a misaligned intervention can put the woman, her partner, and her future baby at risk for physical, emotional, and mental complications if the woman is still active in her eating disorder while going through this experience of trying to conceive.

Dr. Gaudiani states:

> There's a deep societal ill that's being placed upon women which is "stay too small, I'll take all of your money and all of your hope. You don't have to gain weight, you'll be so cute when you're pregnant." We won't really talk about how you're actually caring for yourself and we won't talk about how you might subsequently care for a pregnancy or a child. It feels patriarchal, it feels medically oppressive. It feels damaging. Physicians are an oppressor class for people with eating disorders. . . . Women are always going to take something on themselves—did I do something wrong? It was me. Women are conditioned to respond that way.
>
> What I tell my patients all the time is that upon recovery, they have as good a chance of getting pregnant and sustaining a regular, healthy pregnancy as anyone does. There could be speed-bumps along the way, but that is possible with anyone.[13]

Broaching the subject of an eating disorder and a physician asking about it gives some of the power and control back to the patient and can set them up with a treatment approach that is validating, helpful, and attuned to the patient's specific needs. This helps to reduce shame and secrecy. "I think that medicine has to be narrative," says Dr. Gaudiani. "Patients need to be given the opportunity to share their narrative with their doctors, to blend the stories together (stories of pain and of healing) and make them come to life."

Infertility, Eating Disorders, and Privilege: Advocating for Those Without Resources

Those who struggle with infertility but who are unable to afford the steep price tag of fertility treatment are often left invisibilized. Those who struggle with eating disorders or any form of disordered eating which causes distress to their lives but who are unable to afford counseling or treatment are also often marginalized populations. The cost of fertility treatment can run upwards of $20,000–$40,000 without a guarantee of conceiving a healthy child, although some clinics do offer a partial refund to those who do not have a successful birth after three cycles of IVF. To qualify for this program a patient must fall under certain criteria, such as being age 39 or younger at the time.[14]

Currently only 16 of 50 states in the United States have infertility insurance coverage laws to assist those who qualify for fertility treatment, and four of these states have fertility preservation laws for iatrogenic (medically induced) infertility. Iatrogenesis means any adverse or unintended condition that occurs as a result of treatment for a medical condition. A common instance of iatrogenic infertility is cancer treatment, which can cause the body to go into early menopause and halt egg and hormone production. For a patient who lives in Arkansas, California, Connecticut, Delaware, Hawaii, Illinois, Louisiana, Maryland, Massachusetts, Montana, New Jersey, New York, Ohio, Rhode Island, Texas, or West Virginia and has insurance coverage, they may be eligible for assistance with fertility treatments (with qualifications varying state to state).[15]

This is great news for those that reside in those states and who have insurance coverage and can afford this treatment. What about those who live in the other 34 states, or those who live in any state and cannot afford extensive treatment but so desperately yearn for a family? Most of these patients are in low socioeconomic classes, are nonwhite, unmarried, not heterosexual, or immigrated from a foreign country—populations who are marginalized in multiple other ways by US society. This is where we still have work to do, advocating for these couples and families whose voices are so often disregarded because of their social status. Adoption, which is an option for many couples who struggle to conceive, also costs up to $40,000 without a guarantee of a placement—also out of reach for numerous couples experiencing infertility

Across the country, treatment grants, scholarships, and financing programs for both fertility treatments and adoption are available to qualified couples and families. With the intense emotional distress that infertility can bring to a couple, an additional financial burden of fertility treatments can add more weight to an already stressful situation.

Ciara, a black cisgender married woman, age 29, has been wanting to start a family with her husband, Jevon, who is also black, for the past 2 years. She comes from a big family (six siblings, of which she is the youngest) and has always wanted to have a family of her own, as is normal in her family's culture. Ciara reports regular episodes of binge eating and emotional eating since her adolescence, but she does not fit the criteria for a diagnostic eating disorder.

> We have been trying for a few years to get pregnant. I don't get it. My mama, my grandma, my aunts, my sisters, no one has had issues with it. I would think that I'd be the same. You hear about black women getting pregnant so easily and I have seen it with my friends and relatives. Some of them didn't want to get pregnant or want the child and that makes me angry. I don't know what we're going to do. I've been to the doctor but Jevon and I can't afford all of the tests and procedures they want to do. We certainly couldn't afford IVF. How can people afford that? This has made me just eat more crappy food and then I feel bad because maybe that's why I can't get pregnant? No one seems to understand. I don't know any other black sister who has had issues with getting pregnant—that is what we are bred to do. I think this is a systemic and societal issue, too. You hear mostly about white people being infertile and getting treatment, not about people who aren't white. That's privilege for you.

In a recent study about racial differences in infertility, the authors explore the reasons why white infertility is studied much more prominently than black (in this case) infertility. The authors write:

> The majority of studies on black/white differences in infertility have focused on women who seek infertility treatment. Among these women, black women are significantly different with regard to socioeconomic position and marital status. They have a higher prevalence of some risk factors for infertility such as uterine fibroids and excess weight. They also have a higher prevalence of tubal disease. Overall, this evidence suggests that there are major differences between black women and white women seeking care for infertility. However, whether these differences are present and contribute to increased infertility in black women in the general population is unknown.[16]

Much more discussion and research are warranted on the intersection of fertility and race diversity. Correlation between the rates of treatment for eating disorders in white women and men versus people of color is also skewed. We are shown in the media that most of the people who suffer from eating disorders are white, middle-class heterosexual girls and women. In a study of adolescents, researchers found that Hispanics were significantly more likely to suffer from bulimia nervosa than their non-Hispanic peers. The researchers also reported a trend toward a higher prevalence of binge eating disorder in all minority groups,[17] and black teenagers are 50% more likely than white teenagers to exhibit bulimic behavior, such as binging and purging.[18]

Yet despite similar rates of eating disorders among non-Hispanic whites, Hispanics, African Americans, and Asian Americans, people of color are significantly less likely to receive help for their eating issues.[19]

It is my hypothesis that hundreds of women and men are experiencing infertility and eating disorders but are not reporting them due to stigma, shame, or discrimination, making the rates of these diseases much higher than the current statistics report.

Microaggressions, defined as "a statement, action, or incident regarded as an instance of indirect, subtle, or unintentional discrimination against members of a marginalized group such as a racial or ethnic minority" and macroaggressions, which are "large-scale or overt aggression toward those of a different race, culture, gender, etc." are plentiful and contribute to suffering from these populations.

How Doctors Can Help

Good medical care needs to start with discussion about the generations of power imbalance between physicians and patients, and it is on the doctor to try to name this power imbalance. One way that Dr. Gaudiani tries to navigate this and empower her patients is by always meeting patients fully dressed when she is meeting them for the first time, starting on an equal playing field. She also does not weigh her patients unless she is watching for or treating anorexia, which requires this for health security reasons.

Physicians also can benefit from addressing their own values and biases and working on being less assumptive, and they are encouraged to examine their own internalized size stigma. It's possible to be neutral and Health at Every Size (HAES) focused rather than add to the collective clamor about how unacceptable bodies are outside of a narrowly defined set of criteria. Responses about too much or too little weight gain are not helpful and can lead to shame. Doctors can try to stop judging health by size and shape, but asking "how are you doing, what are you doing?" Stay curious. Asking patients about their goals and values puts the power back in their hands, where it belongs. No one can know them better than the patient knows themselves.

Principles of Health at Every Size work to bring back metabolic and reproductive function and address all parts of a patient's life that may be impacting their emotional and physical health. It includes the following basic components: respect (honoring body diversity in all shapes and sizes); critical awareness (valuing lived experiences and challenging cultural assumptions); and compassionate self-care (finding pleasure and joy in movement and in eating, including listening to the body's hunger and fullness and desire to move in a fulfilling way). HAES is called "the new peace movement" and can have a significant impact in reducing shame in patients with eating disorders or in bodies that do not fit the "cultural ideal."[20]

Patients would benefit from being asked to share if they have a history of an eating disorder or disordered eating; patients may not feel comfortable to advocate for themselves as there is often an overfocus on weight (gain or loss) during pregnancy. This type of screening can give the physician an opportunity to say "let's only do blind weights" and to focus on assessing health from other perspectives. I believe there is a strong need for a standardized assessment tool for eating disorders that fertility clinics and medical offices across the country (and globe) should administer to each of their patients.

Too frequently there is little thoughtfulness by physicians regarding menstrual irregularities in women in larger bodies with binge eating disorder. The assumption often made is that their infertility must be related to PCOS, and weight loss would be the solution. They may miss the opportunity to explore the effect of binge eating on their fertility health. If a woman is in a smaller body, a doctor is more apt to try many interventions to diagnose the source of her fertility issues, pointing back to internalize size stigma and thin privilege. The principles of Health at Every Size work holistically to restore menstrual function from a non-biased perspective, which can reduce stigma and instill deeper trust in the doctor-patient relationship.

How should a doctor navigate a patient who is pregnant or wanting to conceive but who is resistant to recovering from their eating disorder? Keeping them in a weight-inclusive perspective and working with them on clarifying values can help with this also. Does she want to be strong and present enough to carry her toddler around when she is tired? How does she want to look back at the photos and stories from her pregnancy and her child's first few years? What does she want to remember about this time? Helping the patient visualize this can be important and encourage her to move toward a life that really matters to her. Even if the locus of self-compassion for self is dysregulated with the patient, the axis of care and compassion for baby is often strong and intact—this can be an entry point with ED patients, advises Dr. Gaudiani. "Your kid(s) need you. Try to identify what matters more—the eating disorder or your children."

Again, a patient may be terrified that their doctor will judge or shame them if they disclose this inner struggle—or will "make" her get rid of her eating disorder. Knowing that her physician is going to be there for her can instill trust and give the woman a safe relationship that she can explore her ambivalence in. In this situation a doctor could say something like: "I will be here for you no matter what, but may I discuss with you some of the risks of holding on to your ED? What is the narrative going on here? What are your fears of giving it up?" This is work that the woman can be doing with her own therapist, but from the medical perspective it means a great deal to know that her doctor will not abandon her.

Getting Your "Pre-body Baby" Back

When discussing these topics with Dr. Gaudiani, I made a slip of the tongue. As we were talking about body image and pressure to look a certain way during and after pregnancy, I brought up that women feel pressure to get their "pre-body baby" instead of "pre-baby body" back (which is the rhetoric we usually hear).

This invited an interesting discussion—this is what we actually hope women could get! Imagine if we could all go back to the time of our life before we had all of this negative awareness and programming about our bodies and food. I see this intuition with her body in my daughter and feel an overwhelming sense of joy for her and fear for her at the same time. She doesn't have any critical thoughts about her body yet. I hope that she never will, but I also know that we are fighting an uphill battle here and the reality is that she will struggle in some way. But I can be there to continue to give her the message that she is okay and loved just as she is.

Can women get their pre-body baby back? What is this? I'd define it as the experience before you're body-critical, to step back into your own non-self-conscious experience in your body, before you heard any judgmental comments about your own body or others' bodies, before you knew that there was a "standard" that a woman should look like. While we cannot deprogram ourselves as adults, we can work to consciously challenge the thin ideal and societal programming and to encourage our children to accept their bodies as they are.

Clinical Tool: Visualize your Pre-body Baby

See yourself as a baby or toddler, before you had any negative connotations or awareness about your body. Maybe you also bring into your mind an image of your daughter or son. Could you imagine saying to that child the things that you have said to yourself? How would you want to talk with them about their bodies? Can you say these things to yourself?

How to Create a Body-Inclusive and Accepting Home for a Growing Family

Many women and mothers (including myself) experience concern over how to protect their children from experiencing the same struggle with food and body image that they have currently or in the past.

Children of women who have had an eating disorder have genetic factors that may put them at risk for developing a disordered relationship with food, although this certainly is not always the case as many factors contribute to an eating disorder. Our culture has a predominant focus on the thin ideal and supplies young girls and boys with ideas that their bodies need to look a certain way to be accepted, liked, and successful. How can a home environment advocate for a child to learn to listen to and nourish their bodies when they are being socialized to do the exact opposite out in the world? Here are a few ideas:

- Parents can instill an environment for themselves and their children from the feminist and HAES size perspective, meaning that their children have a right to listen to and adhere to what their bodies do and do not want or need, and that all bodies are good bodies, no matter their size or shape.
- Parents can express that home is a safe place to experience hunger, fullness, satiety, body signals, emotions, and so forth.
- Parents can be very aware and cognizant of how they talk about their own bodies at home in front of their children and notice the narrative that they are creating for their children about their own relationship with their bodies. Ask yourself: "Would you say to your child what you say to yourself [about your body, weight, appearance, etc.]?" Try to model healthy self-talk to your children the way you hope they will treat themselves when they are older.
- Parents can help their children understand there are many ways to assess health and wellness other than the number on the scale. They can do this by talking to them about and normalizing emotions, feelings, and needs.
- While parents cannot control or prevent damaging messages that their children may encounter out in society and through social media, creating a safe and accepting home environment is a strong protective factor.
- Parents can spread the message to teachers, fellow parents, and other adult figures in their children's lives about HAES, body acceptance, and the harm that negative body/food/diet talk can have on a child.

Physicians have a strong influence over how safe a patient feels to explore emotional and psychological, as well as physical, factors that may be at play while exploring fertility. This chapter has presented some issues in the doctor-patient relationship that could prohibit adequate intervention in and prevention of eating disorder symptomatology, and outlined some ideas for increasing awareness from a HAES perspective for these issues. More research and work needs to be done to educate medical professionals on how to support their patients' mental and physical health in a destigmatizing way.

Considerations for Therapists

1. What is an example of a microaggression that someone in a marginalized population who struggles with fertility issues may experience? Macroaggressions?
2. What else are doctors missing when addressing fertility issues in women with a current or past eating disorder? How can these be addressed?
3. How can therapists be advocates for their clients struggling with infertility and eating disorders in the interface between them and their medical providers?

Notes

1. Bye, A., Shawe, J., Bick, D., Easter, A., Kash-Macdonald, M., & Micali, N. (2018). Barriers to identifying eating disorders in pregnancy and in the postnatal period: A qualitative approach. *BMC Pregnancy and Childbirth*, *18*(1). https://doi.org/10.1186/s12884-018-1745-x
2. Freizinger, M., Franko, D.L., Dacey, M., Okun, B., & Domar, A.D. (2010). The prevalence of eating disorders in infertile women. *Fertility and Sterility*, *93*(1), 72–78. https://doi.org/10.1016/j.fertnstert.2008.09.055
3. Health at Every Size. (2018). Retrieved from www.haescommunity.org/
4. Bye, A., Shawe, J., Bick, D., Easter, A., Kash-Macdonald, M., & Micali, N. (2018). Barriers to identifying eating disorders in pregnancy and in the postnatal period: A qualitative approach. *BMC Pregnancy and Childbirth*, *18*(1). https://doi.org/10.1186/s12884-018-1745-x
5. Bye, A., Shawe, J., Bick, D., Easter, A., Kash-Macdonald, M., & Micali, N. (2018). Barriers to identifying eating disorders in pregnancy and in the postnatal period: A qualitative approach. *BMC Pregnancy and Childbirth*, *18*(1). https://doi.org/10.1186/s12884-018-1745-x
6. Freizinger, M., Franko, D.L., Dacey, M., Okun, B., & Domar, A.D. (2010). The prevalence of eating disorders in infertile women. *Fertility and Sterility*, *93*(1), 72–78. https://doi.org/10.1016/j.fertnstert.2008.09.055
7. Easter, A., Treasure, J., & Micali, N. (2011). Fertility and prenatal attitudes towards pregnancy in women with eating disorders: Results from the Avon longitudinal study of parents and children. *BJOG: An International Journal of Obstetrics & Gynaecology*, *118*(12), 1491–1498. https://doi.org/10.1111/j.1471-0528.2011.03077.x
8. Kimmel, M., Ferguson, E., Zerwas, S., Bulik, C., & Meltzer-Brody, S. (2015). Obstetric and gynecologic problems associated with eating disorders. *International Journal of Eating Disorders*, *49*(3), 260–275. https://doi.org/10.1002/eat.22483

9. Fogarty, S., Elmir, R., Hay, P., & Schmied, V. (2018). The experience of women with an eating disorder in the perinatal period: A meta-ethnographic study. *BMC Pregnancy and Childbirth*, *18*(1). https://doi.org/10.1186/s12884-018-1762-9
10. Freizinger, M., Franko, D.L., Dacey, M., Okun, B., & Domar, A.D. (2010). The prevalence of eating disorders in infertile women. *Fertility and Sterility*, *93*(1), 72–78. https://doi.org/10.1016/j.fertnstert.2008.09.055
11. Bye, A., Shawe, J., Bick, D., Easter, A., Kash-Macdonald, M., & Micali, N. (2018). Barriers to identifying eating disorders in pregnancy and in the postnatal period: A qualitative approach. *BMC Pregnancy and Childbirth*, *18*(1). https://doi.org/10.1186/s12884-018-1745-x
12. Bye, A., Shawe, J., Bick, D., Easter, A., Kash-Macdonald, M., & Micali, N. (2018). Barriers to identifying eating disorders in pregnancy and in the postnatal period: A qualitative approach. *BMC Pregnancy and Childbirth*, *18*(1). https://doi.org/10.1186/s12884-018-1745-x
13. Gaudiani, J. *The Gaudiani clinic*. Denver, CO.
14. CCRM | IVF Fertility Clinics and Reproductive Family Building Centers. (n.d.). Retrieved from www.ccrmivf.com/
15. Homepage. (2018). Retrieved December 28, 2018, from https://resolve.org/
16. Mellons et al. (Wellons, M.F., Lewis, C.E., Schwartz, S.M., Gunderson, E.P., Schreiner, P.J., Sternfeld, B., Richman, J., Sites, C.K., . . . Siscovick, D.S. (2008). Racial differences in self-reported infertility and risk factors for infertility in a cohort of black and white women: the CARDIA Women's Study. *Fertility and Sterility*, *90*(5), 1640–1648.)
17. Swanson, S.A., Crow, S.J., Le Grange, D., Swendsen, J., & Merikangas, K.R. (2011). Prevalence and correlates of eating disorders in adolescents: Results from the national comorbidity survey replication adolescent supplement. *Archives of General Psychiatry*, *68*(7), 714–723.
18. Goeree, M., Sovinsky, H., John, C., & Iorio, Daniela. (2011). Race, social class, and bulimia nervosa. *IZA Discussion Paper No. 5823*. Retrieved from http://ftp.iza.org/dp5823.pdf.
19. Marques, L., Alegria, M., Becker, A.E., Chen, C., Fang, A., Chosak, A., & Diniz, J.B. (2011). Comparative prevalence, correlates of impairment, and service utilization for eating disorders across U.S. ethnic groups: Implications for reducing ethnic disparities in health care access for eating disorders. *The International Journal of Eating Disorders*, *44*(5), 412–420. http://doi.org/10.1002/eat.20787

    Becker, A.E., Franko, D.L., Speck, A., & Herzog, D.B. (2003). Ethnicity and differential access to care for eating disorder symptoms. *International Journal of Eating Disorders*, *33*(2), 205–212. https://doi.org/10.1002/eat.10129

    Wade, T.D., Keski-Rahkonen, A., & Hudson J. (2011). Epidemiology of eating disorders. In M. Tsuang and M. Tohen (Eds.), *Textbook in Psychiatric Epidemiology* (3rd ed., pp. 343–360). New York: Wiley.
20. Health at Every Size. (2018). Retrieved December 28, 2018, from https://haescommunity.com/

Conclusion

Eating disorders destroy one's ability to think rationally, behave in accordance with one's values, and live a fulfilling life. An eating disorder can have such a tight grip on a person and can affect her so strongly that she may think she cannot, does not deserve, or truly does not want to recover from her illness. And yet a woman may have a yearning to have a family that is so strong that it gets louder than the ED part of her and pushes her to recover fully from the destructive disorder. In this book we have heard from numerous women (and men) who have had an eating disorder, either currently or in the past, and have also desperately wanted to become parents. Many of them fought tooth and nail to get healthy and conceive, whether naturally or through the aid of fertility treatments. Some of them are still fighting—to recover from their ED or to conceive a baby.

What's so interesting to me is the function that an eating disorder has in a person's life. It does not just develop out of nowhere; the terrain must be prepped to set the stage for an ED to come to be. The woman may have incurred verbal, physical or sexual abuse, felt she had a critical parent that made her think she was not enough, may have decided that to be happy, she needed to be thin, and that meant getting as much control of her body as she could. The reasons are numerous that an ED can begin. But for a woman to recover, she has to find meaning in her life that matters more than her ED. She needs to believe that she can push through and feel uncomfortable things in order to love herself. She is called to find some other way of meeting that need that the ED has tried to "help" her meet for so long.

For me, what pushed me through was complete exhaustion of battling my ED and envisioning the family and life that I so desperately wanted one day. Why couldn't I have that too? For so many of the women I have talked to, they have expressed similar desires: to not live in the shadow anymore, to be a role model to her children of what a grounded, self-aware parent looks and acts like. Most significantly, a primary goal of nearly every person I have talked with is to "rewrite their story"; to dedicate themselves to cultivating a secure, safe attachment with their child and to hopefully prevent their children from following in their footsteps.

That is a parent's greatest task: to nurture resiliency, confidence, and perseverance in their children and empower them to fight for radical self-love even in the face of adversity.

It's a battleground out there. Here are some of the words from women I have interviewed, what they might say to someone else going through fertility challenges or struggling to recovery.

Voices From the Trenches: Words of Advice From Those Who Have Been Through It

- "My father used to always tell me that one day my ED is going to be the biggest gift in my life (he struggles with anxiety disorder and panic attacks). That was impossible to even imagine when I spent 7 years absolutely miserable and hopeless. But he was right—and I wouldn't trade those years for anything. Once I got on the other side, I realized that my experience with my ED has given me such a rewarding perspective on life, has added dimension to myself and has made this new life so much more enjoyable—as I know how bad my life can be. I always remind myself that my worst day in this [recovered] life is still 100 times better than my best day in my ED. With a perspective like that, I don't get ruffled by many things and have a solid sense of peace and happiness.

  "I think the most important thing to remember is to not give up on yourself. Ultimately you are the catalyst for recovery. There were so many times I felt like giving up and I am so thankful I didn't. I tried to 'recover' daily for 7 years and I 'failed' daily for 7 years. But I kept trying the next day."
- "I have so much compassion for anyone going through this. None of this is your fault. You are not alone. I would like to encourage people to reach out and talk to one another or seek support. Shame grows in the dark."
- "Try to have the courage to reach out and get the support you need because it really sucks to feel paralyzed by shame and guilt around 'knowing better' while also being responsible on a whole entirely different level for another human being's wellbeing and livelihood. The normal/common self-doubts of being a 'good enough' mom are just compounded."
- "I'd share a passage from Cheryl Strayed's *Tiny Beautiful Things* that affected me to my core. In response to a mother concerned about how her anger would impact her kids, Strayed wrote: 'I don't know, but I do know one thing. When it comes to our children, we do not have the luxury of despair. If we rise, they will rise with us every time, no matter how many times we've fallen before. I hope you will remember that the next time you fail. I hope I will too. Remembering that is the most important work as parents we can possibly do.'"

- "Right now I frankly can say that I'm right there with you. With parenting, time will pass and kids will grow, and that's helping me cope. So perhaps I'd say that it's okay to be disordered at times. Sometimes it's not the right time to focus on it. Again, I know all too well that it's a problem, but there's also only so much time and energy. So perhaps it's okay to just let it be for now."
- "I would say that seeking medical information is so important, and dealing with uncertainty and fear alone isn't worth it. I wish I had asked questions up front, rather than just worried and hoped for the best [ties back to the shame/stigma about opening up to medical professionals about history or current ED]."
- "It's not your fault. It sucks, there is nothing good about infertility, nothing. There will be good days and bad days—days when you're so swallowed by sadness that the idea of living or eating seem impossible. There will be days when it does not bother you and you might feel guilty, and that's ok. I would tell them I understand, and that I know their pain and it's a complicated messy, uncontrollable pain and that trying to fight it or control just makes it bigger. So find people who understand and support you and walk into the fire, sometimes the only way to put out a fire is by letting it burn."
- "Infertility is a tricky thing. It's so individual for each person, yet comparison is an inherent part of this. Comparing to others who have not experienced infertility at all, comparing to others and their different experiences of infertility. I think this leads to an interesting push/pull of wanting to connect to others who have gone through infertility, and then wanting nothing to do with others. Also, there is a very strange/shameful thing that happens when others who you know have experienced infertility get pregnant. I feel so much anger and sadness. But our society tells us this is wrong. It tells us that we should be happy for our friends/people we know that are now pregnant. But that's not how I've felt. It took me a long time to be okay with my feelings of anger towards others who fall pregnant, and sadness for myself that this has not happened for me anymore. And all of this brings SO MUCH SHAME. And secrecy. Because of course we can't tell our friends we feel anger towards them for becoming pregnant. That would be ludicrous. Hence, more shame.

  "*Update*: Now that I am pregnant, I no longer feel like a failure. And this has made me realize that feeling like a failure while enduring infertility is ridiculous. Let me explain. I did nothing different to cause this transfer to do into a pregnancy. It was science. The embryo will work if it is genetically healthy. That is it. It was never my fault that it didn't work, nor was it my 'success' or 'hard work' that this time worked. It's luck and science, that's all. I had zero hope going into transfer. On the day of the transfer my doctor said to me 'Melissa, I want you to think about the fact that our clinic has had a 90% success rate lately. I want to have hope. This makes a difference.' Bullshit. No it doesn't. I basically let what he said go in one ear and out the other. I felt so much hope for our first one and it didn't work. This transfer I felt like there was 99.9% of my body and mind that would not allow me to feel hope. Now that I am pregnant, while incredibly grateful for it, I have intense survivor's guilt. I realize that there are thousands of other people/ couples still dealing with infertility and those questions in their minds of 'will this ever work for me?' It has been difficult for me to allow myself to feel happy about this. Now that I am almost 20 weeks I am allowing myself to feel like it is more real, and plan for this, but at times it is still difficult. I felt like an imposter for the first 14 weeks of being pregnant. Whenever I said 'I'm pregnant' I felt like I was lying. Now that I'm showing it's easier to say it and not feel like an imposter, but it still feels surreal at times.

"I want to say something to others that I think is not said: YOU DO NOT HAVE TO HAVE HOPE. I know this sounds crazy, but hope killed me. If one more person said to me during this process 'just have hope' I was going to lose it. I did lose it. If you have no hope, that is okay. Your thoughts and your mindset do not make a difference in your outcome. If it feels good to have hope, have it. If it feels like you will be more devastated to have hope, let it go."

- "Even if someone struggles with getting pregnant, it is ok to have all kinds of feelings about having a child. One can pray and do all they can to get pregnant and then struggle with the pregnancy itself or postpartum (or both!) and that doesn't need to be made more difficult with feelings of guilt or shame about not loving pregnancy or parenthood at times. We are all human and can feel many conflicting feelings and that is OK."
- (to a parent with pregnancy and ED): "Take it one day at a time, minute to minute when necessary. 10 months is a long time and it can be overwhelming to think of it all at once. In taking it moment to moment, day to day, it can give a sense of ease and a possibility to get through it rather than feeling like it's impossible. Also, don't isolate yourself. Healing is done in community and there's nothing more reassuring and validating than a 'me too'—connect with others who may be in the same place or who have gone through it."
- (to a new parent with ED): "Breathe. Be sure to take care of yourself—determine what are your absolutely necessary daily self-care practices and ensure you do them. Certainly sleep, eating regularly, staying hydrated, and some kind of body movement are the basics, but don't forget about them! Then, what else do you need? I need to get sunshine and a shower daily to truly feel like myself, so I make sure to do these every single day. Remember, you are a new person now so you may need to establish new self-care practices as a result."

- "To anyone experiencing infertility, I want to send the most heartfelt hug. Infertility (after alcoholism) was the most difficult and challenging time of my life. But wow, I've seen so many people create their own families in their own unique ways and it's amazing."
- "Your body is a gift. It is so incredibly magical to feel the growth of a small person inside of you and to be able to bring that into the world. For me, it was so healing. And also a constant reminder of what kind of body-message I want to send to my children."
- "I would say that the smallest bit of progress is just as important as any big milestones. I recommend bookmarking inspirational and touching stories to read when you're frustrated and feel hopeless about the body you're in. The topic doesn't have to be physical appearance, it can be about anything that makes you feel grateful for other thing(s) that are going well in your life. I am more appreciative of my thighs when I remember that many do not have the opportunity to walk on their own two legs."
- "It will become necessary to create a different relationship with your body where the focus becomes expanding, in my case, instead of shrinking. I have learned to do this physically as well as emotionally. Seek support. Have compassion for yourself. The pain can be excruciating at times, and it's hard not to want to wage war against your body again. Love yourself through it. Be gentle and patient with yourself."
- "Both infertility and an ED are isolating and the isolation can feel compounded when they're occurring simultaneously. People without ED's struggle as new parents to adjust to the demands and change of focus from yourself and/or your marriage/spouse to a new person who needs everything from you. It's terrifying and wonderful. Get help if you need it—being a 'good parent' means taking care of yourself so that you can be at your best for your child."
- "It's hard as f*$@! Ask for a lot of help . . . even before [getting pregnant or giving birth], and let folks know what they may see from you that would clue them in to the fact you may be struggling."
- "I felt shamed and not heard by my medical team. These experiences deepened my feelings of shame and I wish I would've been stronger, known more, and advocated for myself more. I definitely feel that my mistrust of and shame regarding my body had an impact on my ability to advocate for myself."
- "The pain and fear come in waves. Weathering the storm of this situation is impossible to do alone. There are so many questions and uncertainty that the majority of the people in your world will never be able to understand. I feel the most important thing to do is to find someone to talk to about everything. Be as open and real with that person as possible. And preferably find someone who has personally experienced/studied disordered eating. It's amazing how an outside,

unbiased person who will be sensitive but also real with you can change your entire perspective on the situation.

- "I hope you can stop comparing yourself to photoshopped models and Instagram fitness accounts. UNFOLLOW THEM. Get them out of your phone, out of your head, out of your life. We need to stop forcing our bodies to conform to our idea of what beauty looks like. Instead, honor what your body wants. If it needs ice cream, eat the dang ice cream and don't look back. If it needs a day, a month, a year away from the gym, honor that. Throw your scale away and eat food. Lots of it. And please, by all means, don't go down the road I did. I learned the hard way so you don't have to. You are more than the size of your body! You are YOU, so love that, flaunt that and live the life God intends you to live, which I can promise you, is not one full of celery and treadmills."[1]

Thank you so much to each person who helped contribute to this book. Thank you for opening up your souls so that others who are walking their own path can find consolation and hope. I am grateful to be in your company and am not quite sure who I would be without it.

We have much more work to do to shed the light about the intersection of infertility and eating disorders. Advocacy around setting up a more thorough and universal and weight neutral assessment process of eating disorders at fertility clinics and OB/GYN medical offices is warranted, perhaps including the development of an evidence-based assessment tool that becomes part of standard procedure in medical offices across the country.

Note

1. Made Me Infertile. (2018, November 13). Retrieved from www.kiwiandcarrot.com/fitness-made-me-infertile/

Bibliography

Agras, S., Hammer, L., & McNicholas, F. (1999). A prospective study of the influence of eating-disordered mothers on their children. *International Journal of Eating Disorders*, 25, 253.

ART Success Rates. (2018, September 11). Retrieved December 28, 2018, from www.cdc.gov/art/artdata/index.html

Astrachan-Fletcher, E., Veldhuis, C., Lively, N., Fowler, C., & Marcks, B. (2008). The reciprocal effects of eating disorders and the postpartum period: A review of the literature and recommendations for clinical care. *Journal of Women's Health*, *17*(2), 227–239. https://doi.org/10.1089/jwh.2007.0550

Behavioral Change Models. (n.d.). Retrieved from http://sphweb.bumc.bu.edu/otlt/MPH-Modules/SB/BehavioralChangeTheories/BehavioralChangeTheories6.html

Benoit, D. (2004). Infant-parent attachment: Definition, types, antecedents, measurement and outcome. *Paediatrics & Child Health*, *9*(8), 541–545. https://doi.org/10.1093/pch/9.8.541

Benson, E. (2003, November). *The many faces of perfectionism*. Retrieved from www.apa.org/monitor/nov03/manyfaces.aspx

Brach, T. (2012). *Radical acceptance: Awakening the love that heals fear and shame*. London: Ebury Digital.

Brown, B. (2015). *Daring greatly: How the courage to be vulnerable transforms the way we live, love, parent, and lead*. London: Penguin Life.

Bulik, C.M., Hoffman, E.R., Holle, A.V., Torgersen, L., Stoltenberg, C., & Reichborn-Kjennerud, T. (2010). Unplanned pregnancy in women with Anorexia Nervosa. *Obstetrics & Gynecology*, *116*(5), 1136–1140. https://doi.org/10.1097/aog.0b013e3181f7efdc

Bye, A., Shawe, J., Bick, D., Easter, A., Kash-Macdonald, M., & Micali, N. (2018). Barriers to identifying eating disorders in pregnancy and in the postnatal period: A qualitative approach. *BMC Pregnancy and Childbirth*, *18*(1). https://doi.org/10.1186/s12884–018–1745-x

CCRM | IVF Fertility Clinics and Reproductive Family Building Centers. (n.d.). Retrieved from www.ccrmivf.com/

Costin, C. (2017). *8 keys to recovery from an eating disorder*. New York, NY: W.W. Norton.

Domar, A.D., & Kelly, A.L. (2004). *Conquering infertility: Dr. Alice Domar's guide to enhancing fertility and coping with infertility*. London: Penguin Books.

DSM-5. (2013). *Diagnostic and statistical manual of mental disorders*. Arlington, VA: American Psychiatric Association.

Easter, A., Treasure, J., & Micali, N. (2011). Fertility and prenatal attitudes towards pregnancy in women with eating disorders: Results from the Avon longitudinal study of parents and children. *BJOG: An International Journal of Obstetrics & Gynaecology*, *118*(12), 1491–1498. https://doi.org/10.1111/j.1471–0528.2011.03077.x

"Fitness" Made Me Infertile. (2018, November 13). Retrieved from www.kiwiandcarrot.com/fitness-made-me-infertile/

Fogarty, S., Elmir, R., Hay, P., & Schmied, V. (2018). The experience of women with an eating disorder in the perinatal period: A meta-ethnographic study. *BMC Pregnancy and Childbirth*, *18*(1). https://doi.org/10.1186/s12884-018-1762-9

Freizinger, M., Franko, D.L., Dacey, M., Okun, B., & Domar, A.D. (2010). The prevalence of eating disorders in infertile women. *Fertility and Sterility*, *93*(1), 72–78. https://doi.org/10.1016/j.fertnstert.2008.09.055

Galhardo, A., Pinto-Gouveia, J., Cunha, M., & Matos, M. (2011). The impact of shame and self-judgment on psychopathology in infertile patients. *Human Reproduction*, *26*(9), 2408–2414. https://doi.org/10.1093/humrep/der209

Genogram. (2018, December 24). Retrieved December 30, 2018, from https://en.wikipedia.org/wiki/Genogram

Health at Every Size. (n.d.). Retrieved December 28, 2018, from https://haescommunity.com/

Home. (n.d.a). Retrieved December 28, 2018, from https://connect.asrm.org/home?ssopc=1

Home. (n.d.b). Retrieved December 30, 2018, from www.brenebrown.com/

Homepage. (n.d.). Retrieved December 28, 2018, from https://resolve.org/

Kimmel, M., Ferguson, E., Zerwas, S., Bulik, C., & Meltzer-Brody, S. (2015). Obstetric and gynecologic problems associated with eating disorders. *International Journal of Eating Disorders*, *49*(3), 260–275. https://doi.org/10.1002/eat.22483

Koubaa, S., Hällström, T., & Hirschberg, A.L. (2008). Early maternal adjustment in women with eating disorders. *International Journal of Eating Disorders*, *41*(5), 405–410. https://doi.org/10.1002/eat.20521

Lacey, J.H., & Smith, G. (1987). Bulimia nervosa: The impact of pregnancy on mother and baby. British Journal of Psychiatry, 150, 777.

Lai, B.P., & Tang, C.S. (2008). The negative impact of maternal bulimic symptoms on parenting behavior. *Journal of Psychosomatic Research*, *65*(2), 181–189. https://doi.org/10.1016/j.jpsychores.2008.04.003

Leeune, J. (2016). *20 science-based recommendations for therapy with highly self-critical or shame-prone clients*. Retrieved December 30, 2018, from www.actwithcompassion.com/20_science_based_recommendations_for_therapy_with_highly_self_critical_or_shame_prone_clients

Lemberg, R., & Phillips, J. (1989). The impact of pregnancy on anorexia and bulimia nervosa. *International Journal of Eating Disorders*, *8*, 285.

Linna, M.S., Raevuori, A., Haukka, J., Suvisaari, J.M., Suokas, J.T., & Gissler, M. (2013). Reproductive health outcomes in eating disorders. *International Journal of Eating Disorders*, *46*(8), 826–833. https://doi.org/10.1002/eat.22179

Mccabe, M. P., & Ricciardelli, L. A. (2004). Body image dissatisfaction among males across the lifespan. *Journal of Psychosomatic Research*, *56*(6), 675–685. doi:10.1016/s0022-3999(03)00129-6

Mercer, W.M. (1997). *Infertility as a covered benefit*. Retrieved December 28, 2018, from https://resolve.org/infertility-101/what-is-infertility/fast-facts/

Micali, N., Simonoff, E., & Treasure, J. (2011). Pregnancy and post-partum depression and anxiety in a longitudinal general population cohort: The effect of eating disorders and past depression. *Journal of Affective Disorders*, *131*(1–3), 150–157. https://doi.org/10.1016/j.jad.2010.09.034

Michelmore, K., Balen, A., & Dunger, D. (2001). Polycystic ovaries and eating disorders: Are they related? *Human Reproduction*, *16*(4), 765–769. https://doi.org/10.1093/humrep/16.4.765

Morgan, J. F, Lacey, J.H., & Sedgwick, P.M. (1999). Impact of pregnancy on bulimia nervosa. *British Journal of Psychiatry*, *174*, 135.

Mysko, C., & Amadeï, M. (2009). *Does this pregnancy make me look fat?: The essential guide to loving your body before and after baby*. Deerfield Beach, FL: Health Communications.

National Center for Health Statistics 2006–2010. (2018, December 19). Retrieved December 28, 2018, from www.cdc.gov/nchs/nsfg/index.htm

National Women's Health Resource Center. (n.d.). Retrieved December 28, 2018, from https://rarediseases.org/organizations/national-womens-health-resource-center

Neff, K. (2015). *Self-compassion: Stop beating yourself up and leave insecurity behind*. New York: William Morrow.

Olwyn, G. (2011, November 11). *Reproductive health I: Fertility & pregnancy*. Retrieved December 30, 2018, from https://edinstitute.org/paper/2011/11/11/reproductive-health-i-fertility-pregnancy

Pasquali, R. (2006). Obesity and androgens: Facts and perspectives. *Fertility and Sterility*, *85*(5), 1319–1340. https://doi.org/10.1016/j.fertnstert.2005.10.054

Perfectionism (psychology). (2018, December 24). Retrieved from https://en.wikipedia.org/wiki/Perfectionism_(psychology)

Priel, B., & Besser, A. (2000). Adult attachment styles, early relationships, antenatal attachment, and perceptions of infant temperament: A study of first-time mothers. *Personal Relationships*, *7*(3), 291–310. https://doi.org/10.1111/j.1475–6811.2000.tb00018.x

Reba-Harrelson, L., Holle, A. V., Hamer, R.M., Torgersen, L., Reichborn-Kjennerud, T., & Bulik, C.M. (2010). Patterns of maternal feeding and child eating associated with eating disorders in the Norwegian mother and child cohort study (MoBa). *Eating Behaviors*, *11*(1), 54–61. https://doi.org/10.1016/j.eatbeh.2009.09.004

Ruggeri, A. (2018, February 21). *Future: The dangerous downsides of perfectionism*. Retrieved from www.bbc.com/future/story/20180219-toxic-perfectionism-is-on-the-rise

Russell, G.F., Treasure, J., & Eisler, I. (1998). Mothers with anorexia nervosa who underfeed their children: Their recognition and management. *Psychological Medicine*, *28*(1), 93–108. https://doi.org/10.1017/s003329179700603x

Sadeh-Sharvit, S., Levy-Shiff, R., Arnow, K.D., & Lock, J.D. (2016). The interactions of mothers with eating disorders with their toddlers: Identifying broader risk factors. *Attachment & Human Development*, *18*(4), 418–428. https://doi.org/10.1080/14616734.2016.1164201

Secondary infertility: Why does it happen? (2017, February 08). Retrieved December 30, 2018, from www.mayoclinic.org/diseases-conditions/infertility/expert-answers/secondary-infertility/faq-20058272

Six Tips for Handling Survivor Guilt. (n.d.). Retrieved December 30, 2018, from www.psychologytoday.com/us/blog/how-be-yourself/201711/six-tips-handling-survivor-guilt

Statistics & Research on Eating Disorders. (2018, September 14). Retrieved December 28, 2018, from www.nationaleatingdisorders.org/statistics-research-eating-disorders

Statistics & Research on Eating Disorders. (2018, September 14). Retrieved from www.nationaleatingdisorders.org/statistics-research-eating-disorders

Stewart, D.E., Raskin, J., Garfinkel, P.E., MacDonald, O.L., & Robinson, G.E. (1987). Anorexia nervosa, bulimia, and pregnancy. *American Journal of Obstetrics and Gynecology*, 157, 1194.

Tribole, E., & Resch, E. (2012). *Intuitive eating: A revolutionary program that works*. New York: St. Martins Griffin.

Wallace, K. (2013, November 20). *'Pregorexia': Extreme dieting by pregnant women*. Retrieved December 30, 2018, from www.cnn.com/2013/11/20/living/pregnant-dieting-pregorexia-moms/index.html

Weiss, H. (2015). *Hakomi mindfulness-centered somatic psychotherapy: A comprehensive guide to theory and practice*. New York: W.W. Norton & Company.

What causes amenorrhea? (n.d.). Retrieved December 28, 2018, from www.nichd.nih.gov/health/topics/amenorrhea/conditioninfo/causes

Index

Note: Page numbers in *italics* indicate a figure on the corresponding page.

abortion 16, 44, 67, 127
abuse 20, 140; alcohol 67; laxative *see* laxative abuse; substance *see* substance abuse
acceptance and commitment therapy (ACT) 120
active eating disorders and pregnancy 41, 58–59
adiponectin 37
adoption 68–69, 132–133
adversity 141
allowing the pain as a clinical tool 120–121
amenorrhea 13–14, 18, 42; hypothalamic 13, 61; and infertility 29, 42
androgens 15, 37
anorexia nervosa (AN) 13–16, 19; atypical 131; binge-purge type 3, 94, 117; lifetime 42; and miscarriage 37; and unintentional pregnancy 42; restricting type 3
anorexia nervosa and attempting to conceive [personal stories] 27–30, 38–40
"anorexic identity" 43, 66
anovular infertility 18
anxiety 94; over appearance 104, 112; and childbirth 77; depression and 17–18, 21, 80, 118; during meals 22; and perfectionism 105–106, 114, 121; and pregnancy 47, 49, 52, 56, 64, 66–67, 76; over having a second child 38
anxiety, struggling with [personal stories] 3–9, 39, 40, 70, 73, 80–82, 85–90, 94–99
anxiety disorder 77, 116
Apgar score 18
appetite 18, 37, 52, 59, 66
attachment *see* parent-child attachment; postpartum attachment
avoidant/restrictive food intake disorder (ARFID) 3, 13

"baby weight" 111
back problems during pregnancy 53
bariatric surgery 124
belly 49, 66, 113
"belly stories" as a clinical tool 46–47, 49
Bermudez, Ovidio 111–112
binge eating disorder (BED) 2, 3, 5, 14–16, 91; atypical 131; awareness of 129; and fertility 135; generational impact 96, 107; media influence on 112; and pregnancy loss 36–37; among minority groups 134; and shame 115, 125; and unintentional pregnancy 42
binge eating disorder and attempting to conceive [personal stories] 40–41, 43
binge eating disorder outside diagnostic criteria and infertility [personal stories] 133
binge cycles 22, 64
binge drinking 42, 67
binge/purge pattern 42–43, 65, 67, 70, 90, 93
birth control 60, 67, 118, 124
birth trauma 43, 44, 77–78, 94
birth trauma [personal stories of] 77–78

black women with eating disorders 133–134
blind weights 46, 135
bonding 69, 72, 92; as distinct from attaching 99; with baby 78, 81; with fetus 82; with child 83; maternal difficulties with 17; *see also* mother-child bonding
bonding instinct 83
"body ideal" 71
body image 48, 71; in preadolescents and teens 71–73; postpartum (after pregnancy) 64, 69, 90; during pregnancy 47–48, 64; and social ideals 103; *see also* pregnant body image
Brown, Brené 102, 110–111, 126
bulimia nervosa (BN) i, 3, 5–6, 12, 131; and abortion 127; and attachment issues 93; exercise 113; features of 14–15; and PCOS 37; and people of color 134; and risky behavior 42; and unintended pregnancy 16
bulimia and attachment issues [personal stories of] 98–99
bulimia and shame [personal stories of] 64, 83, 107–108
Bye, A. 126, 128, 129

"caveman brain" 14, 36, 127
clinical tools: allowing for the pain 121; "belly stories" as 46–47; family pregnancy and body image genogram 73; identity web 84; "letters to my baby" 78, 99; metaphor 65; self-compassion 111; visualization 85; working though guilt to acceptance 76; working with shame and infertility 110
conception (and ED) 10, 25–26, 76; clinical tools pertaining to 30–34; complexities of 49; costs 132; desire to 8; and PPD 90; and privilege 132–134; statistics 2; struggles to 12, 89, 131, 140; triggering potential 66; women in recovery 26–28; *see also* infertility; miscarriage; physicians; pregnancy loss
constipation 45, 52
Costin, Carolyn 25
Curan, Thomas 105

Diagnostic and Statistical Manual of Mental Disorders, Fifth Edition (DSM-5) 13, 15, 59, 64, 112, 131
depression 116, 90; and androgens 37; and anxiety *see* anxiety; and infertility 116; and perfectionism 106; and shame 119; postpartum *see* postpartum depression
depression and struggles with conception [personal stories] 41, 91–93
diabetes 37, 64
diarrhea 45
diet 30, 43, 46, 57; fad 107; healthy 118; plan 64, 89; putting children on 72; restrictive 62; vegan 109; *see also* orthorexia
Diet Mentality 55–56
diet pills 4
dietary: factors 37; guidelines 41
diet/binge mentality 64
dieting 15, 20, 30, 54; and binge eating 91; extreme 108
dysthymia disorder 116

eating disorders (EDs) 3–11; barriers to identifying 128; maternal 21; during pregnancy 47–48; relapsing 43
eating disorders and attachment [personal stories] 82–83
eating disorders and infertility [personal stories] 117–119
eating disorders and pregnancy [personal stories] 43–44
eating disorders and pregnancy loss [personal stories] 44–45
eating disorder identity 17, 48, 70
ejaculatory disorders 19
embryo 2, 28–30, 35, 41, 49, 142
emotional mood swings and hormone fluctuations during pregnancy 53; *see also* postpartum mood disorders
endocrine disorders 37; *see also* polycystic ovary syndrome
endometriosis 37, 38, 108, 109
estrogen 19, 30, 60, 71
exercise: disordered relationship to 19, 20, 25, 28, 30; and children 72; excessive 36, 67; healthy 63, 118; lack of time for 91, 92; as maladaptive coping mechanism 113; militant 57; orthorexic

60; over- 41; planning 89; preoccupation with 93
exercise addiction 53, 67, 81, 112
exhaustion during pregnancy 53

fallopian tubes 29, 38
fat-shaming 125
fear 17, 25, 26, 34, 46, 83; of gaining weight 95, 112, 114; and giving birth 80; of judgement 127; of losing custody 96; during pregnancy 38, 49, 52, 58, 64, 69; mindset 14; and shame 136, 142; and stigma 130, 142; subconscious 102; *see also* anorexia; pregorexia; survivor's guilt
fear, pregnancy, and ED [personal stories] 9, 12, 27–29, 77, 85, 88
fear-shame cycle *114*
fertility and ED 1–10, 22, 25–26; current research on 12–15; effect of eating disorders on 16–18, 27–29, 41–45; emotional factors impacting 125; and "fitness" 61–62; loss of 69; medical complications; and race 134; return of 63; struggles 70, 80, 89, 106; treatments 78, 121, 127–129, 131–135, 140–141; *see also* infertility; in vitro fertilization
fertility challenges and ED [personal stories] 141–145
fetus 36, 46, 49, 127, 130; bonding with 78, 82; pregorexia and 112
fight, flight or freeze 14
Flett, Gordon 103, 106
Fogarty, S. 47–48
food cravings or aversions 53, 61
forgetfulness, memory loss 53
frozen embryo transfer (FET) 41

Gaudiani, Jennifer 42, 116, 126, 131, 134
genogram as a clinical tool 73–75, *74*
gonadotropin-releasing hormone (GnRH) 14
guilt 41, 69; and anxiety 81; during pregnancy 46, 47, 55–56, 58, 64; maternal 83, 85, 90; and mental illness 99; and miscarriage 44; and perfectionism 121; and self-doubt 39; and shame 22, 28, 34, 35, 82, 102, 112–113, 126, 141; *see also* survivor's guilt

Hakomi therapy 32
Health at Every Size (HAES) 15, 115, 126, 134–135, 138
heartburn 45
highly sensitive person (HSP) 5
Hill, Andrew 104, 105
hyperemesis gravidarum 54
hypertension 37
hypothalamic amenorrhea 13, 61
hypothalamus 14
hypothyroidism 61
hysterectomy 109

iatrogenic infertility 132; *see also* infertility
identity web as clinical tool 84–85, *86*
impulsive personality traits 16, 37
infertility 1–2, 10; clinical tools 30–34; and eating disorders 3, 12, 22, *31*; idiopathic (unexplained) 29; *see also* miscarriage; primary infertility; secondary infertility
infertility and ED [personal stories of] 36, 38–41
insulin resistance 37
insurance 2, 124, 132
insomnia/sleep issues during pregnancy 9, 53
International Committee for Monitoring Assisted Reproductive Technologies (ICMART) 1
intrauterine insemination *see* IUI
intuitive eating: during pregnancy 54–55; ten principles of 55–58
in vitro fertilization (IVF) 2, 28, 35, 29, 52; costs of 132, 133
in vitro fertilization and ED [stories of] 41, 117, 120, 125
IUI 28, 29, 41, 52, 121

laxative abuse 36, 41, 45, 107, 113
leptin 18, 37
"letters to my baby" as clinical tool 78; 99–100

magical thinking 5, 42, 44, 58
male infertility 18–20
mature maternal age 12
medical community, what it needs to know to support clients 124–128, 134–136; advocacy and privilege 130–134; barriers to identifying eating disorders 128–130; body-inclusivity 137–138

menses 17, 43
menstruation, menstrual cycle and ED 5, 13; irregularities 15, 16, 18, 37, 67, 124; loss of 41, 42; and PCOS
mental illness 42, 99
metaphor as a clinical tool 65–66
Micali, N. 41, 42
microaggression 134
miscarriage and pregnancy loss 34–37
mood disorders *see* postpartum mood disorders
mortality 90
"mother" as an identity 48
"mother" as a role 9, 43
mother's body 35, 46, 53
mother (with ED) and child 14, 16–17; *see also* parent-child attachment; postpartum attachment
motherhood 10, 19, 107, 108, 110; and infertility 38, 22; longing for 44; perceptions of 67, 73, 102; *see also* postpartum attachment
motherhood ideal 108
morning sickness 45, 53, 54
Mysko, Claire 111–112
nausea during pregnancy 53; *see also* morning sickness

Neff, Kristin 119–120

Obama, Michelle 35
obesity 2, 15, 16, 36–37, 41
oligomenorrhea 18
oocyte abnormality 37
orthorexia 59–65
orthorexia and pregnancy [personal stories] 60–65
osteopenia 60, 61
otherwise specified feeding and eating disorder (OSFED) 3, 13, 16
ovulation disorders 38, 42

parent-child attachment in recovery 97
parent-child attachment with ED [personal story] 97–99
perfectionism 4, 7, 10, 90; and anorexia 106; and anxiety 95, 121; progress not 57; rise in 105; and shame *see* shame
perfectionism and ED [personal stories] 73
polycystic ovary syndrome (PCOS) 2, 15; definition and characteristics 37–38
post-traumatic stress disorder (PTSD) *see* PTSD
postpartum anxiety (PPA) 66–67
postpartum attachment 17, 20–22, 44; and motherhood 80–81; with current ED 47–48, 93–94
postpartum attachment with current ED [personal stories] 94–97
postpartum depression (PPD) 24, 38, 44–45, 50; and anxiety 66, 73, 81, 87–88
postpartum depression and anxiety [personal stories] 73
postpartum mood disorders 87–91, 97, 114
postpartum mood disorders and ED [personal stories] 88–93, 98
postpartum relapse 44, 58, 59, 82, 83, 90, 94, 95, 108
pre-baby body 64, 82, 111, 136
"pre-body baby" 136
preeclampsia 64, 90
pregnancy: and active eating disorder 41–45; intuitive eating during 46; triggering impacts on ED recovery 45–46
pregnancy with ED [personal stories of] 43–45, 80–81
pregnant body image 47, 59
pregnant body image and ED [personal stories of] 47–48
pregorexia 64, 111–112
pregorexia and pregnancy [personal stories] 114–116
primary infertility 38, 41
probes in mindfulness 32–34
progesterone 32, 39
PTSD 38; and birth trauma 77; in pregnancy 75–76
PTSD and pregnancy [personal stories of] 75, 76–77
purging 15, 45

Rasmussen, Katie 105
recovery [from an eating disorder] 25–26; five stages of 26; and the desire to get pregnant 27–30; and the experience of fertility issues 53–55
recovery and fertility issues [personal stories] 81–82
recovery and parent-child attachment 97–99
recovery and perfectionism 106–107

recovery and perfectionism [personal stories] 108–110
recovery and pregnancy [personal stories] 57–58
relapse [of ED] 17, 20, 26, 29, 45–46; postpartum *see* postpartum relapse
remission [of ED symptoms] during pregnancy 4, 59, 90, 127
restriction (food) 45
Rice, Kenneth 103
risky behavior 42

Sadeh-Sharvit, S. 21–22, 93
secondary infertility 38–41
self-acceptance 10, 22, 84, 102, 108
self-care 7, 9, 59, 81, 135
self-compassion 32, 68, 70, 84, 90, 111, 118
self-compassion as a clinical tool 111
self-concept 94, 97
self-confidence 58
self-criticism 48, 87, 103, 118
self-damaging 49
self-destruction 65
self-devaluation 118
self-doubt 39
self-esteem 20, 21, 37, 53, 107; and dieting 55
self-harm 107
self-isolation 37
self-judgement 12, 48, 99, 119
self-kindness 120
self-management 129
self-preservation 127
self-protection 40
self-soothing 91
self-worth 75, 105
shame 2–6, 8, 10–12, 13; and infertility 22, 25, 27–31; in men 18, 20; and perfectionism 10, 102–120; and relationships 116; and secrecy 102; underlying factor of 44; *see also* miscarriage
shame and perfectionism [personal stories of] 107–100
"shame container" 31
"shame proneness" 119, 121
shame resilience therapy (SRT) 110
Smitt, Natalie 95–96
sperm production disorders 19
"state shame" 119, 121
stigma 19, 97, 99, 103, 124, 126; mental illness 96, 127; miscarriage 35; weight 15, 18, 125, 128
Stone, Elizabeth 52
Strayed, Cheryl 141
stretch marks and growth of hips/breasts during pregnancy 53
substance abuse 35, 120
survivor's guilt 38, 75–76, 143

testosterone 19, 20, 37, 71
"thin ideal" 122
thyroid disease 2
trauma 110, 116, 124; childhood 27; emotional 32; *see also* birth trauma; post-traumatic stress disorder

underfeeding 22
unintentional parent 25, 66–71
unintentional pregnancy 16, 17, 42, 54, 58, 77, 127
uterine conditions 38

visualization as clinical tool 85–87

weight stigma 15, 18, 19, 126, 127, 130
weight gain during pregnancy 53; clinical overfocus on 124, 135
working through guilt as a clinical tool 76
working with shame as a clinical tool 110–111